P9-BYL-623

I Beat Cancer
50 People Tell You How They Did It

Awareness Publishing
Oxnard, CA

First Printing June, 2003

ISBN 0-9721678-0-3

LCCN 2003091563

Disclaimer

This book is for educational purposes only. It is not a substitute for a trained physician. The reader is advised to see a doctor for any physical problem.

The publisher cannot take responsibility for the use and application for any information presented herein. There is no guarantee of cancer prevention or survival.

For information on any of the clinics discussed in this book, order the new, updated Fourth Edition of *Third Opinion*, by John M. Fink, due Fall 2003. This is an international directory of alternative therapy centers for the treatment and prevention of cancer and other degenerative diseases. It includes names, addresses, phone numbers, web sites, methods of treatment, approaches, costs, glossary of terms, regional listings and more.

For more information on how to order this book, contact:
Square One Publishing
115 Herrick's Road
Garden City Park, New York 11040
(877) 900-BOOK

You can also get information on the clinics on the Cure Research Foundation's website at www.cancure.org.

Contact Information

Contact information for most of the people who have shared their stories in this book is available at http://www.awarenesspublishing.com/contact.

Table of Contents

Foreword

Today is January 28, 2003. Finally, I feel ready to write my story. Every story in the book is finished but mine. I have been trying to write my story since I first realized the great need for a book like this. This is the book I hoped to find when I was diagnosed with breast cancer in 2001. This project has taken about 9 months, and there have been great moments putting it together. I have spoken to many wonderful people who have taught me so much.

I just got off the phone with my doctor's office. They were calling to give me the results of an extensive list of blood tests taken last week. As I sat in anticipation of the results, I remembered again how scary cancer can be. As the nurse reads me the results and tells me everything is as good as it gets, I feel myself breath a deep sigh of relief. Yippee.... I get to stay alive (at least for now)... I get to raise my kids, love my husband, learn, grow and contribute.

How lucky I have been to be able to speak to so many heroes of cancer! When I first asked people who had beaten cancer if they would be kind enough to tell their story and help others, I thought we were putting together a winning list of protocols for beating cancer. I expected that the book would be all about what clinic or what vitamin or regimen they attributed to their success.

As the stories started coming in I realized that almost every story told about a protocol that was different from others. Some people did juicing, some drank Essiac tea, some used immune building products... and, astounding to me is the fact that all of these people are well today.

A question kept coming up in my mind. With so many unique protocols, what is the commonality that made the difference between life and death for each of them? Although there is no one answer, I put together a list of common characteristics I noticed in my contact with this group of survivors. Although I could not say any of these is the total answer, I believe there are some things worth looking into. I hope further research will be conducted to see what role these qualities play in someone's survival.

1. A STRONG desire to live. An attitude that no matter what they have to do, they are not going to die right now. They feel they still have much to experience and death is just out of the question at this time.

2. They have taken the responsibility for their health into their own hands, finding out as much as they can, getting more opinions, as opposed to giving it to someone else to handle. ("Don't tell me about it, just zap crackle and pop me so I can go on with my life the way it is!") In Europe they are starting to take a *cut and wait* approach, rather than further compromising the immune system with chemo and radiation therapy. Take the tumor burden out of the body, and let the immune system get on with its job.

3. They realize that the cancer is a call, and they pay attention to the call. They change how they eat and most importantly how they think. Most people seem to go through a change in viewpoint as a result of their diagnosis. They express great gratitude for their lives and a desire to help others. They get forced into letting go of the things that seemed so important before, like worries of the future, and instead find a new *"live in the moment"* awareness. Taking time to smell the roses is an often heard remark.

4. They make a stronger spiritual connection. They surrender to a higher power. They stop trying to struggle through life and force things to happen. Once you have experienced a life threatening illness you realize that everything is out of your control. You could die at any time, and certainly as the expression goes, "No one gets out alive!"

I have seen that cancer has dramatically improved these

people's lives. It changes ones' narrow perspective, and opens one up to realize that this is such a short journey, and there is no guarantee of any future. We need to be in every moment fully and appreciate the many gifts that life gives us.

Bliss Page

Bliss Page
Breast Cancer

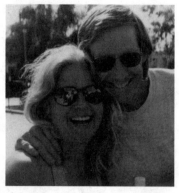

The diagnosis of cancer has to be the best thing to ever happen to me in this life, although it sure didn't seem like it when I found out. It was 2001, and I had been feeling pain in my right breast. I decided to go to the local hospital and get a mammogram. Since I was always in good health and a vegetarian and considered myself *health conscious*, I really never considered cancer even a possibility.

After the needle biopsy, I had the lab fax the pathology report to me at home. As I stood over the fax machine I saw the word *carcinoma*. That was it. That's where the fear started and it gathered momentum for months.

I started looking up every word of the report on the Internet to learn something about it. I had never really thought about it. It doesn't run in my family and I was only 46.

I found an excellent breast surgeon, and agreed to a lumpectomy and sentinel node biopsy (in which they preserve the breast by removing just the tumor and the first few lymph nodes under the arm for further diagnosis).

The lab report after the surgery had 3 basic pieces of information:

    1) The Grade: Mine was one of the most aggressive — Grade 3. 2) Margins: Was all of the tumor removed?

Simply... NO 3) Lymph nodes: Was there any malignancy detected in the nodes? Yes, two of the four were positive for malignancy.

So, I took that report to the Internet and could see by some simple charts that on average I had about a 12% chance of surviving 5 years. The fear of death was so intense, I might have died from fright... Hmmm! Could the fear of *impending death* ultimately cause it? Could the minds' fear actually accelerate the body's demise?

The surgeon recommended a full mastectomy and removal of the rest of the lymph nodes under my arm. This would be followed by chemotherapy and many doses of radiation. I would also be a good candidate for Tamoxifin.

The bad news kept coming. My mother was diagnosed with liver cancer within a week of my diagnosis. She came to live with us, but died on her 4th day with us. I watched first hand what cancer can do.

I struggled with what to do.... After much soul and Internet searching, I realized that I would decline what the medical community had to offer. I felt I had to become my own doctor of sorts and treat myself. My feeling was that if the cancer should take me, at least I did everything I could to continue living. Simply stated, I took the responsibility for my health, instead of putting it in the hands of others. I would accept the help of others, but I would be responsible. In fact, that is how I've always lived my life.

My very loving and committed husband of 15 years was with me to support and help heal me. I feel so blessed to have him in my life.

I found a web site that specialized in alternative cancer cures: www.cancure.org. I met a wonderful and informative woman, Melinda Wiman (who, incidentally, helped edit this book). She gave me some references of people who might be able to help me. I researched a number of people and clinics and finally decided on Dr. Chappell in Ojai, California. He put me on a detoxing and cleansing protocol. After a few weeks of carrot juice, colonics, vitamin C, exercise, and other treatments to boost the immune system, I started feeling terrific.

I have had a number of blood tests and scans and they all show that I am cancer free. I am so grateful for this experience, because it made me look at my life in ways I had never done before.

Probably the best thing about cancer is that it made me look at death. Our culture hides death from us. I used to have to turn away if I saw a dead animal in the road. I used to say "if I die" when I spoke about my own death.

So, I started asking, "What is death?" I have come to realize some things that have calmed my fear of cancer. When I was in my 20's, I had two out-of-body experiences. Once I was in a hospital on an operating table when suddenly I was near the ceiling looking down at the doctors, and my body on the table. I could clearly hear them talking about a fishing vacation. The second event occurred when I was driving my car and the accelerator pedal got stuck as I was merging onto a completely stopped freeway with nowhere to turn. I believed that my life was ending. Pictures of my past started flashing before me. I was looking down on my body from above my head and saw the side of my face from a direction I could not have seen in any mirror. Suddenly I looked at my hand as it turned the ignition off. I was watching as if someone else was doing it, since turning off the ignition hadn't even occurred to me.

These events made me realize that the essence that I am is much more than my body. I realized that if "I" was my body then how could "I" be watching it and seeing it as just a body. I really felt no special attachment to it. I knew that it was the body I had been inhabiting, but that was all.

I had realized conceptually that we are here only temporarily in these bodies. Faced with a life threatening illness I surrendered more deeply to this concept. My new awareness was one of peace. If birth and death are not the beginning or ending, but are only transitions, then what's the problem? I realized the only problem was, that I didn't want to leave my life *story*. In the story, I play a wife and mother and many other parts, but none of the parts is the true essence which occupies this body. I realized the intense vastness of life.

I can see a gradual letting go of my story, and a more deepening of who I really am. I am appreciating every moment as precious. When I find myself thinking of the past or fearing the future, I take a deep breath and relax, knowing that NOW is really all there is. I live as fully in the NOW as I possibly can... now.

I believe illness and dis-ease are the result of our unconscious thoughts. The mind is always coming up with problems to think about. I notice that all of these problems have a physical connection to them. When I am thinking of a problem my body is picking up on those thoughts. It believes there is a real event occurring even if it's only in thought. I notice how the body contracts with pain, and the breathing becomes shallower. The body is always listening with deep awareness. It believes what the mind tells it. Is this an ironic fact of our current state of evolution — That the childish, fearful mind is senior to the deep awareness of the body?

I now use the mind to know unconditionally that my body's health is excellent, and that it will live a long life. There is nothing to fear since everything is unfolding as it needs to with great perfection. I am so very grateful for the many gifts with which this *dis-ease* has provided me. If you are dealing with a similar condition, I hope you too will come to appreciate it for the many new awarenesses it can bring!

Finally, I would suggest a book that has helped me to understand more deeply who or what I am, as opposed to the story I am living in this body. It is called *Practicing The Power of Now* by Eckhart Tolle. It can change your life.

PAUL LEVERETT
BRAIN STEM GLIOBLASTOMA

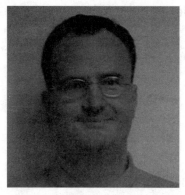

I will try to make my point, but I like to tell stories so I will just try to get clear up front. If you or a loved one is fighting cancer you need to go in with your eyes wide open. Doctors are really smart people, but they are just people. They should not be put in the exalted position that our society has put them in. They don't know everything. They are just men and women. They are highly trained technicians. Most mean well. Some are just trying to get paid.

You need to educate yourself. You need to be involved in your own healing. If you just sit back and let the hospitals and doctors take over and do whatever they think best, then don't be surprised if the results are far less than you expected.

Get a second opinion. I know you have heard this before. It is true. Two heads really are better than one. Get your head in the equation as well. The Internet is a great source. Obviously, "buyer beware." There are a multitude of books out there. Do some research.

This became obvious to me when my initial oncologist wanted to try the same old therapies on me that had so far not worked for anyone else in my condition. In my business, we were forced to figure out how to put drilling rigs to work in conditions they were never designed for. When the customer asked us to do this we put a bunch of engineers on the task and tried to figure out a way. This *can do* attitude was not readily apparent at my first hospital and oncologist. Don't keep doing the same things over and over again expecting or hoping for different results.

I had a certain disease. Brain stem Glioblastoma Multiforme. They had a list of approved therapies to treat me. That was that.

Engineers and doctors are a lot alike. Both are intelligent. Both do great things. Build bridges, cure diseases. Very analytical. Great. But after working with engineers for nearly 20 years, it is easy to see that they are just people like you and me. They don't know everything. They are not smarter than everyone else. Smart. Just not smarter than everyone else. This obviously applies to doctors as well. Smart. Sometimes brilliant. Not smarter than everyone else.

Okay, enough said on that. I hope you get my point. You must do your homework. You need to be informed. Do not leave this fight only up to your physician. He/she is only human. Say a prayer, educate yourself, and trust your intuition.

God bless you.

THE DIAGNOSIS

It was maybe mid-April 99. I was in Vietnam negotiating a difficult contract. The symptoms were not really evident, but were there. The skin on my forehead was slightly numb. I put it off to too much jogging and the sun in Vung Tau. It just wasn't that annoying. A few days later a good friend of mine was jogging next to me at the club in Jakarta and thought I may have had a mild stroke. What he saw was my left eye opening wider than my right eye. I put it off to my lazy right eye. Anyway, we would be in Singapore soon and I would get a full check up. I had been noticing numbness in my feet after a hard workout on a Stairmaster. Also, my left hand would get a little tingling after jogging for a while. I would see a cardiologist in Singapore in May. I would just schedule the appointment right after our region meeting. No worries.

On top of all the minor worries or symptoms I just didn't feel at the top of my game. My jogging was getting harder, not easier. I thought I might even have some exotic Asian bug. Something was just not right.

Just before our meeting in May, I made a trip to Myanmar (Burma) as we had no presence there and there was a job prospect to check out. Before dinner with the client I needed a nap. Dinner was difficult as the client was French, the meal was duck, and of course, there was wine and cheese. Indigestion. Apparently another symptom of my condition. Another symptom I just blew off.

Back to Jakarta. Prepare for Singapore. Then off to the meeting. Five days of meetings helping the region management plan for up coming jobs and possible contracts. It was a good meeting. I exercised every day. My wife (girl friend at the time) joined me. Jennie worked for an airline (Cathay Pacific) at the time. Jennie was able to make her schedule flexible. I traveled all over the Far East, including Hong Kong. So even though Jennie lived in Hong Kong at the time and I in Jakarta, we were both able to manage our schedules enough so that we were together at least 2 to 3 weekends per month. I was trying hard to convince her to marry me. She just didn't like my job. She didn't like the schedule I kept. That was all about to change.

I had worked nearly 20 years for the oil well drilling division of Schlumberger. I was the marketing manager for the region in the Far East. Our area stretched from Bangladesh to Japan and Sakhalin Island including Indonesia and Australasia. Big area with lots of flying. The best 2 years so far of my nearly 20 years. I was enjoying myself. The operations secretary at our office in Singapore (Julie) had helped to organize the meeting and had scheduled me with the doctor I wanted to see. The doctor was an American cardiologist living in Singapore. The hospital was Mt. Elizabeth. At the end of the region meeting I had things I wanted to do relating to what I had learned from the meeting. I nearly cancelled the appointment with the doctor. Jennie convinced me to go see him. It was about 2 pm. The cardiologist checked me out. I explained the symptoms. He said my heart was as strong as a bull's and thought I may have carpal tunnel syndrome, if anything. Therefore, he would like me to go see a neurospecialist in the same building. He called the doctor and the doctor fit me in right away.

In the meeting with the neurospecialist, he said that before we could have an intelligent conversation he needed me to do an MRI. This was a bit over the top, he explained, but he would just like to be sure of what he was talking about. So, he called the MRI center in the same building and made me an appointment straight away. Their efficiency was starting to worry me a little. Even by Singapore standards things were moving really fast.

Halfway through the MRI, the technician came in and said that the radiologist had seen something and wanted to give me an injection to try and highlight it. Fear and loathing. She injected me with the isotope and continued the MRI. We finished up about 5 pm and went back to the cardiologist. He explained that the MRI was a little extra but they just wanted to be clear. I should come back in the morning about 9 am to visit with the neurospecialist.

That night we went to dinner and went to the night safari. They have this zoo where you walk in a tropical forest among the animals. Kind of cool to be just across a canal from a Bengal tiger. I was worried and did not feel very good about things. MRI's just mess you up. I think the radiation affects you. I obviously felt worse.

The next day we went to the Singaporean neurospecialist. I didn't wait long and almost went straight into the man's office. My scan is there on his view box. It seems there is this huge white dot in the middle of the scan. Things are not right.

I sit down. The doctor tells me straight away that they have found the problem. You have a tumor on your brain stem. Very abrupt and to the point. He tells me there is nothing they can do for me in Singapore and that I needed to go back to the USA. He noted that Houston, Texas was a good place to go. They may be able to help there. The cardiologist wanted to see me before I left, so I go see him. Okay. Good luck. Good bye. I had paid for the session the day before. This day they didn't need any money.

I walked into the hallway and told Jennie that I was dying. She was shocked and held my hand. We went to see the cardiologist. He tried to make me feel better. Told me that there were all kinds of radiosurgery techniques now. Go home now. Good luck. Good bye. He also did not need to get paid that day.

I went back to the hotel Mandarin Oriental. Sat down and cried with Jennie. Called my boss, Mike, also my friend. I told him I had just been diagnosed with a brain tumor. He came over immediately. Arranged for Jennie and I to go back to Houston immediately. First class. This was Friday May 21 1999. I turned 40 on April 19, 1999. I had just hit the stride in my career. I wanted to get married to Jennie. I never imagined I would want to give my heart so completely to a woman. Things were going well for a change. I had just been run over by a freight train. This was surreal. How could this be happening? The next day Jennie and I were off to the airport. Jennie for Hong Kong. Me for Jakarta. I had double vision on the way to the airport. This thing was coming sooner rather than later. Time was obviously running out. I dropped Jennie off at the Cathay terminal then I was off to Jakarta. Both of us went to pack up our lives. I had not lived in the US for nearly 20 years. Jennie never. Fear and loathing.

Back in Jakarta I went to the office and started to get the stuff I did not want left behind. I knew I wasn't coming back. Searched the Internet in all the usual sites for my condition. Things didn't look good. It seemed the consistent prognosis was 44 to 72 weeks from diagnosis for a malignant tumor in the brain stem. Then death. We still didn't know if this thing in me was malignant. Apparently there wasn't much hope that it wasn't. Hoping for a miracle.

Back at my apartment. I called Walter and Dan, two good friends I worked with. Gave them the news. Arranged dinner that night at my place with Mike, Dan, and Walter. Had some wine. Played some poker. Said good bye to my friends. Mike had walked his dying father up the stairs to his bed for the last time as he had died of cancer, so he knew a little about what I was going through. He was trying to help. Compassion came naturally. Walter came over the next day to help me pack. Walter and I were posted in Nigeria together. Walter is a huge man. He could hardly keep from crying. Huge man. Huge heart. Walter, the maid, and myself packed up that day. Pretty good job. We got everything. I was ready to leave it all. Without Walter and the Indonesian maid (Santi) this would never have been accomplished. The next day I was off to the USA via Hong Kong to pick up Jennie.

I called my younger brother and sister and let them know. This ruined their day in more ways than were immediately obvious.

Mike had called people we both knew that were in the right positions to help in Schlumberger Houston. When we arrived there was a car to pick us up and take us to an apartment rented for me by the company. Not bad. A softer landing. As you will see throughout this story my company and the insurance company they fund really did right by me. I was surprised. I expected much less. I am a bit cynical. It is still hard for me to believe all the things they did for me. Schlumberger took care of me.

My brother, sister, Jennie and I all moved in together in a 2 bedroom apartment rented for me by the company. I thought this may be good, as I did not know how much help Jennie would need, never having lived in the US. I did not know how disabled I would be or how soon.

From Jakarta I had sent my US-based physician an

email explaining my problem and asking for his help getting me in front of the appropriate doctor to help me. I had an appointment the day after I arrived the US. This neurosurgeon had a good reputation and wasted no time in telling me he could do nothing for me and telling me that I needed to be at M.D. Anderson Cancer Hospital. He knew the head of the neurosurgery department there and would help me get an appointment. He didn't take any money either.

SURGERY

M.D. Anderson needed me to pay for the first meeting in advance before they would even book an appointment. However, they didn't want the money from me, they wanted it from my insurance company. Of course they wanted to be connected to the deep pockets. Luckily my insurance company moved quickly and we were ready to go in a day or so. This is a company-funded insurance plan for employees administered by a firm out of Brussels, Belgium (European Benefits). So we were dealing with a time difference. This did not matter once we made that first connection.

At the meeting with the head of the neurosurgery department at M.D. Anderson, he recommended a biopsy to determine exactly what type of tumor we were dealing with. It just may be benign, very slow growing, or something else. All very unlikely, but we needed to know what we were up against. The two choices for biopsy were 1) a needle through the top of the brain down to the brain stem to extract some of the tumor, or 2) place me on my side, cut open the left side of my head, drain out my brain fluid, let the brain sag down so that the brain stem is visible, then remove what tumor can be removed and go from there. The surgeon recommended option 2. We chose option 2. At least get something done while you are in there.

Before all this got going Jennie and I got married in a little Hispanic wedding chapel on a Saturday. Then we applied civilly on Monday. You have to wait 2 days in Texas. We also needed a will.

By the 2nd of June I was on the operating table. The surgery took about 7 hours. The tumor was inoperable, but they removed an outcropping to the left of my brain stem. The surgeon told my wife, while I was in recovery, that the biopsy would take 2 or 3 days to analyze, but he felt it was a glioblastoma grade 3, judging by what he could see and by my symptoms. He also felt this tumor was slow growing, as it seemed to have been there for awhile. Anyway, the surgeon broke it down for Jennie: The tumor could be benign or grade 1, but it did not look like it so we would not hope for that. Grade 2 would mean a slow growing tumor and I could probably live up to 5 years. Grade 3 would mean I may have as much as 2 years, and a grade 4 would mean less than a year. The end would come quick. He thought that due to my symptoms I could very possibly have a grade 3 tumor. We would know in a few days.

It took me 2 days to get out of the hospital. We went back for the biopsy result. I guess there is just no good way of giving bad news. We had already waited a while to get into the examining room. Once there our doctor kept walking by our examining room never looking in. Finally the surgeon arrives. Grade 4. Next step is for you to be turned over to an oncologist who would quarterback the rest of my treatment. The prognosis has been explained to your wife. However, you are 40, strong, so you never know. Sorry. Good bye.

After surgery Jennie had to fly back to Hong Kong. Quit her job. Pack up her life. Close down everything. Get out of her lease. Round trip in 4 days. I was on pins and needles. Immigration and all. That's all we needed. Some pinhead in immigration "just doing his/her job."

I had been searching frantically on the web for some alternative. Diet, supplements, another type of therapy. Nothing seemed very promising. I ran across Burzynski and antineoplastons, but my brother, being from Houston, told me of his troubles. However, he may not even practice any more. Forget about it. It was just a scam. Some woman in my brother's office was telling my brother to be sure and get proof of any success claimed by Burzynski before I spent any money there. Okay. Seems hopeless. I also did not ask MDA for proof of any success before I went there. As if that means anything.

MDA lined me up with a psychiatrist. I guess she was there to assist me along my final path. I remember that she was an atheist. Some spiritual help she was. I guess I was deserving of this. I had led a fairly secular life over the last 25 years. Attending this meeting with the psychiatrist and me were Jennie, my brother, and sister. Anyway, this meeting quickly deteriorated into a meeting all about my sister's anger and her problems. The psychiatrist did tell me in front of my sister that this was my time and that I may need to make some decisions about who should be included. For this clarity I am grateful. Anyway, the psychiatrist's assistance for my final journey was not welcome. I had other plans.

BETRAYAL and CLARITY

In addition to what we had been going through, my sister had gone AWOL with money from some of my investment properties. It turns out she had gone to all of my tenants (about 75% occupied apartments at the time) the morning of my surgery and had the tenants write their checks that month to her so she could get me cash in the hospital. I didn't get any cash and I never saw her after that. She also had the other 25% of my apartments rented out in her name, telling me they were empty while I was overseas. Now that I was back she (they) became desperate. My brother had done everything he could to defend her. There was something not correct here either but we needed my brother's help and so we didn't dig any further. Things just *smelled* wrong. My brother was obviously involved in the scheme. I just could not concentrate on this now. The freight trains just kept coming.

ENLIGHTENMENT

I found another way. One night I just collapsed. I couldn't take dying this way. I did not want to die. Things were just getting good. I was in love. I wanted to live. I went to our bedroom and got on my knees and started praying to God. I had not prayed in 25 years. I begged the Lord to guide me. Give me peace. Heal me. I needed a miracle.

I started searching and praying for a miracle. It seemed nothing could help me. Less than 1% chance of survival is what I was faced with. This was no option. I prayed constantly for guidance, wisdom, and knowledge. The Lord started to work in my life. In small ways. Intuitively I just knew it. How to get over that less than 1% hurdle?

I felt things were happening in my life, which was the work of the Holy Spirit. Jennie, my friends, my company, insurance, no financial worries really as the company was backing us. I just had this intuition that I wanted to go to Burzynski. Jennie felt that way too. It was strong and consistent. Against all advice from the people around us that were *advising* us.

I had been trying to figure out a way to end it all and still keep my insurance in tact for Jennie. When I told Jennie, she held my hand and asked me to try. To pray. To stay and be with her. I got a new fight in me. I was going to die trying.

About this same time, some friends visited. They encouraged me. Said they were praying for me. We went to church together. Michel and Tommy have been incredible support for me. Tommy went to Lourdes in France and got Holy water from there for me.

I don't know about Holy water, but I do believe in the power of prayer and support. A person's touch. I remember when Michel just grabbed my head and me and cursed my tumor and told it to get out of his friend's head. These things mean a lot to someone terminally ill. It meant a lot to me.

My friends really supported me. I was a little blushed at how people from all over the world came to my aid and support. People from all different faiths, beliefs, and walks of life. We are all indeed human. For this I am forever grateful. I have been blessed.

RADIATION

When can we get the radiation started? I was pushing for it, but was told I would need to wait 2 weeks. I don't think we have 2 weeks. It was a low dose due to the location of my tumor. Did not want to get too rough. I might die. Go figure.

Finally I got an appointment to be fitted for the radiation machine. I thought we were ready to go. I went for my appointment that was so difficult to get, only to find my radiation oncologist was on vacation. His assistant baby doctor was there to help me fill out all the disclaimers. If I died doing this treatment they were not accountable. Etc., etc. Great. Cover your ass. Can we hit the microwave now? I told this young doctor to get the lead out, that I was sitting here behind the 8 ball and he wants me to wait for this prima donna to get back from his vacation while I've got the *alien* growing in my head.

Apparently a GBM doubles in size every 2 weeks. Nice. This joker is on vacation and I've got the *alien* ready to pop out of my head. "Will some one get Sigourney Weaver here for me?" So, we get measured that day. I think it was a Thursday. We started our 6 weeks of treatment the next Monday.

Each Monday you were supposed to go visit your radiation oncologist to see how things were going. Well the first Monday he was still on vacation so we went to visit him the second Monday. The follow up is scheduled the same day as your radiation session, 6 hours later. So you can come back downtown and spend another 3 hours messing around at MDA. We show up at 1 pm for our appointment. We had already been there at 7 am. Maybe this doctor has something positive to say. Well about 3 pm we get invited in to the examining room. Another 15 minutes or so this arrogant little vacationer comes in and spends about 5 minutes with me. I ask him if he knows anything about Burzynski. He does. He is very condescending but does claim to know that Burzynski's treatment does have some efficacy. Very negative. Anyway, that was it. I never went back for another Monday waste of time. I even encouraged other patients to boycott this stupid waste of time. We are sheep. I think there was one that followed my small rebellion.

Knowing what I know now I would not have wasted my time on this old, outdated, and antiquated treatment. A waste of time in my opinion. The hospitals are still just trying to get those big machines paid for again.

BURZYNSKI

I was on the web every day and night. I prayed constantly with Jennie. We went to mass every day. Repeated the prayer to St. Jude every day several times a day. There must be something. There are a lot of people out there ready to take your money. The only thing besides supplements and nutrition that held some promise in my opinion was Burzynski. I was on a very strict detox diet. I was doing coffee enemas. I was taking 20,000 mg of Vitamin C every day, as well as IP6, bovine tracheal cartilage, and CoQ10. All therapeutic doses. I drank my own urine for 6 weeks. I was taking a whole list of brain-related supplements and herbal remedies.

There are supposed to be some brain specific herbs. Not everything crosses the blood brain barrier. One needs to do homework and as they say "exercise caution." You could die. And then?

I went to healing touch where the practitioner tries to align your energy flow so that your body can heal itself. We even went to visit a shaman. Probably the most suspect of anything I did. The point is you need to do everything you can. Don't just wait on the doctors. Because in my opinion they just don't know what to do for terminal cases.

If you do the research you will see what I mean.

I only took supplements that apparently crossed the blood brain barrier. Go to Amazon.com and you can search for all kinds of books on fighting cancer. Fighting cancer is an individual journey. We all have our own path. I was also meditating and doing affirmations every day several times a day. There are several books by O. Carl Simonton on meditation. John Kehoe has some good thoughts on affirmations. Affirmations attracted me the most. The belief that your subconscious mind can heal. Train your subconscious mind to do any thing you want. Use that brain power to heal. Seemed that nothing else would work.

The web is a great tool, but beware. There are a lot of folks out there just trying to separate you and your money. They don't care if you are sick or not.

Just before the end of radiation Jennie and I went to interview with Dr. Burzynski. We both had our censors on full. I am strongly inclined to base decisions on intuition. When I can, I try to marry both intuition and analytical analysis. Too much of one or the other and you won't make the right decision. I looked Dr. Burzynski in the eye and asked him about my case. He told me precisely the type of chemotherapy MDA would offer me (MDA had yet to recommend a chemo-poison, but when they did, Burzynski was right). Burzynski had analyzed my blood work, and reviewed my chart to date. He told me that antineoplastons had only a 30% chance of interacting with my tumor. If it did interact with my tumor, there was a 50% chance that antineoplastons could stop the tumor. Let's see: even if he was exaggerating a little, any number over 1 is already a huge increase in my current odds. Okay. Let's roll.

This was all wonderful news. However, my doctors, my brother, the radiation oncologist friend of my best friend from High School and University (who is a doctor in Birmingham), had told me that Dr. Burzynski was a charlatan! Who was right?

Jennie and I were praying. We had been given no hope at MDA. No hope anywhere. Nutrition, supplements, meditation, affirmation, on and on. No hope. Blood brain barrier. No way. You are dead. Get with the program.

We decided to give Burzynski a shot. It would just be 6

weeks. If the antineoplastons did not work, then we would be released. Another dead-end.

We went for a follow up appointment with our oncologist at MDA. The radiation had reduced my tumor by 20%. The chemo offered was as Burzynski had predicted. Just a couple of weeks before that there was a 3 page email of options from my oncologist. No trials however. I did not fit any criteria.

So we were going to try again what had so far not worked in any condition similar to mine. Great. What is that about expecting different results by doing the same things over again? Anyway, we told this doctor that we were thinking of going to Burzynski. He responded that this would not hurt his feelings. His tone was a little condescending. Whatever.

We were off to Burzynski. Burzynski had a few success stories we were welcome to speak with. I didn't bother. I thought it might not be real. And I did not want the negativity of a suspicious mind working against me just in case I did not believe the survivor. MDA had no survivors with my condition. My attitude was that if I was going to die anyway at least die trying. But still the last thing you want is to die being taken advantage of. Let's see.

The FDA requires one to wait 2 months before starting Burzynski's protocol if you have done some other standard course of therapy. Just in case that other therapy may work. With a tumor that doubles in size every 2 weeks that is really valuable time for someone with not much. I'm sure in their wisdom the FDA is protecting the public. Really?

So Jennie and I went to a meditation camp in Santa Barbara, California hosted by Dr. O. Carl Simonton. There they teach you how to find your path to healing or dying. They encourage you to live, but if it is time to die they try to help you come to terms with that. I still could not get past the going peaceful part. I wanted to fight this S.O.B. inside my head and I would not go peacefully. My affirmations always attacked my tumor. I would guide and encourage my immune system to kill my cancer. They teach this method of fighting cancer.

Once we got started at Burzynski, the tumor had grown back 11%. There was some discussion between my oncologist at MDA and what Burzynski was saying as I was still doing my MRI's at MDA. However, this stopped after we got a call from my oncologist to say I should stop Burzynski as something was going wrong with the tumor. Really? It was growing to the cerebellum or some such stuff. This call came through my brother and so I really doubt the accuracy of the call. Jennie called the MDA oncologist back to understand what he was talking about but he never returned her call. My brother really did not want me to follow the Burzynski protocol. ("Why spend more money? It would mean less money for those left behind.")

Whatever. I remember Jennie and I decided that if MDA had nothing new to offer, we would just continue with Burzynski. By the summer of 2000, my tumor had reduced by more than 54%. No hope of making it out of 1999 alive and now this unstoppable tumor was actually reducing.

My tumor was officially declared in complete remission December, 2000. I stayed on the treatment until September, 2001. I now get an MRI and PET scan every six months. My tumor is dead and continues to reduce in size.

I believe the most effective parts of my healing were Dr. Stanislaw Burzynski's antineoplastons, my faith in God, and my dedicated and determined wife (Jennie) who basically made sure I did my treatment as prescribed. She was also part of God's plan for me.

SHDEMA GOODMAN
BREAST CANCER

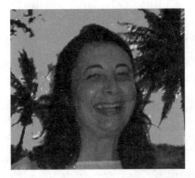

I know the terror of cancer first hand. I have been diagnosed with cancer three times. By the third bout, I just couldn't face another round of surgery and chemotherapy, which had left me so debilitated that I wasn't even able to make a phone call. I felt that if I went to the hospital again, I was going to die. Instead, I decided to give myself three months to practice what I had been teaching for many years as a psychologist, using the latest scientific research in mind/body medicine and ageless wisdom. At the completion of my self-healing program in 1995, the doctor examined me and said, "A miracle has happened, your cancer is gone!" "It's not a miracle, doctor," I replied, "I have been practicing self healing for an hour three times a day." "You must write about it," he responded. "That is too stressful, you write about it," I muttered to myself.

Cancer is predicted soon to become the number one killer. Clearly, the current treatment is not working. Even the very mention of the word *cancer* evokes fear because, for most people, it means death.

What I have learned from mind/body medicine is that surgery and drugs only remove the symptoms of cancer, not the cause. Unless the cause is healed, cancer will reappear. Experience has shown me that our self-sabotaging attitudes about ourselves are like poison to the body, weakening and eventually disabling our body's immune system, creating cancer. Changing these toxic attitudes to healing decisions enables the body to begin to heal itself. Symptoms are messages from the body that our toxic attitudes are having a detrimental effect on the body. My own triumph over cancer and working with those challenging cancer all around the world has taught me that cancer is the result of a denial of our inherent goodness and worthiness, and an identification with not being good or worthy enough. We then become filled with fear and doubt — rather than the love and joy of our true self — and the body begins to break down.

In 1992, right after my initial diagnosis with breast cancer, I took a vow that if I made it, I would devote my life to help erase sickness, pain and suffering from humanity. I have just finished writing my book, *The Goodman Guide in Preventing or Reversing Cancer and Other Diseases in as Little as 30 Minutes a Day,* which describes this program in self-healing. This is in partial fulfillment of my vow. In this book, readers are shown how to find the psychological and spiritual blocks that stop the flow of life force in the body which ultimately causes cancer, and how to dissolve these blocks so the body can heal itself. I draw on my own journey of how I denied my needs when I made unconscious decisions against myself. I show people how to reconnect with their goodness and find their heart's bliss and passion for life that naturally brings them joy and healing. People learn how to heal themselves on all levels — physically, emotionally, mentally and spiritually.

My research into biofeedback in the early 1980s showed me how the mind affects the body. In addition, numerous validated research findings confirmed the ability to reverse physiological disorders with the mind. I understood that there is a physiological response in every cell of the body to every thought we think.

In 1984 I founded and directed the Biofeedback, Psychology and Stress Management Center in Livingston,

New Jersey. I had a large private practice and helped thousands of people solve a variety of problems from emotional to physical disorders. I became known for my expertise in reversing psychosomatic disorders using Gestalt therapy, biofeedback and self-hypnosis. The beneficial combination of these modalities led me to develop a program that helped alleviate many physiological disorders, such as hypertension, ulcers, arthritis, rheumatism, headaches and back pain. All kinds of aches and pains were successfully treated. I also dealt with anxiety, depression, phobias, relationship problems and other psychological disorders on a daily basis. This combination of modalities was helpful in all the cases I dealt with.

When cancer appeared in my life, I started exploring the possibility that the body/mind connection theories would also apply to cancer. I studied extensively, researching articles and participating in many programs and seminars. I learned about the field of scientific research called Psychoneuroimmunology or PNI. Broken down into its parts, here is what Psychoneuroimmunology means: *Psycho* is how thoughts, *neuro* affect the nervous system and *immunology* is how it affects the immune system. Our thoughts affect our nervous system, which then affects our immune system.

WHAT TOXIC ATTITUDES DO TO THE BODY

The latest research in PNI shows that our negative thoughts and emotions slowly destroy our immune system until disease occurs. These negative thoughts and emotions solidify into attitudes that are toxic to the body and make us sick. Strong sarcastic, skeptical, pessimistic attitudes create energy blockages which stop the flow of vital life force energy (hormones, chemicals and nutrients that are usually carried to all parts of the body) depleting the immune system until disease starts. If these destructive attitudes are not changed, the discomfort grows and the sickness gets worse, eventually killing us.

From my experience working with cancer patients all over the world using the program in my book, it is the psychological and spiritual blocks that prevent us from radiant health. Having also studied numerous ancient healing traditions for over 30 years, I have learned that psychological issues that have not been resolved create internal tension. That tension blocks the flow of the life force in the body/mind systems. These blockages are the reason for the diseases that develop in the physical body.

I have tried numerous alternative program, vitamins, diets, juicing, herbs — you name it, I did it. But my cancer kept marching on, until I dropped everything in my life and practiced the self-healing program on a daily basis, by myself. Within three months the 4 cm tumor shrank down to 2 cm. My swollen lymph nodes returned to normal and the pain I had throughout my body diminished. Eight months later I had regained perfect health.

A woman from London, who was diagnosed with terminal bone cancer, had been told by her doctors there was nothing they could do to help her. She healed using the program that is in the book and it is four years now that she is in good health.

A physician from New York, who was diagnosed with colon cancer practiced just one exercise in the book, for five to ten minutes three times a day, and his cancerous tumor disappeared in one week, making his scheduled surgery unnecessary.

A young man with AIDS was told that he had a few days to live. He walked home from the hospital, attended my seminar and two years later he is in radiant health. This is the email he just sent me:

"I think about you all the time, and every morning when I meditate I send my gratitude to you. You really inspired me to try to live one more time and I am. I have a permanent *piece* of a house in New Mexico and I live in New York now. My health is great ... my T-cells are almost above normal and my white blood cells are above normal. You should see me; you wouldn't even recognize me."

These are but a few of countless people who have learned how to heal themselves. If I could do it, so can anyone. I am a simple person.

KIM MORENO
BRAIN STEM GLIOMA

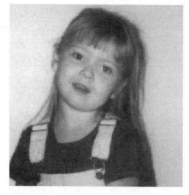

This story is about my daughter, Tori Moreno. She was diagnosed at the age of 7 weeks old, with a Brain Stem Glioma. We were given no hope with conventional treatment, and were told to take our daughter home and prepare for her to die within 2-6 weeks. Prepare for her to die? That *course of treatment* did not come with any instructions and emotionally left us stifled with fear. How do you do this? How do I prepare to watch my child die? I had no idea what to do, where to go or where to search for the mere strength to handle this. We took her home and started to try to prepare for what was ahead of us.

Tori was put on Decadron, and we immediately watched our little angel begin to suffer. She swelled up like a balloon, was irritable and starving and quite frankly, I don't know how her heart survived the strain. Mine was barely making it, she was so much stronger than I could ever imagine being. After several weeks of *mourning*, we decided to hit the Internet for any information we could find. We ran across a treatment that was being offered in Houston, Texas by a Dr. Stanislaw Burzynski at the Burzynski Research Institute. It was a clinical trial involving a non-toxic type of gene therapy, something we had never heard of, something our doctors told us was *quackery*. We contacted the clinic and were told the Doctor had great success with Tori's particular type of tumor and chances of survival would be around 33%. That was a huge increase from the 0% chance we had been given, and we decided it was worth looking into. It didn't take much to convince us. Just a few phone calls to people in similar situations where they themselves or their child had been given another day of life.

Tori started treatment at the age of 3 1/2 months. The doctor was confident he could help, he was just unsure if he had time. She was to be placed on a 24 hour IV therapy, that we were to learn how to administer at home. Within two weeks of being on the treatment, her symptoms decreased. She could blink her left eye, which she did not before. Her left eye tracked better than before and her facial palsy started to decrease. She managed to remain on treatment under close supervision and her first MRI showed a 20% decrease. Within 4 months, she was completely weaned off of Decadron and was still managing the treatment incredibly well. Her tumor to date is down 87%. She is on a capsule form of the treatment and continues to progress every day. A miracle? A divine intervention? Absolutely. That is what she is for sure. She is now 4 1/2 years old. Walking, talking, running ... living the life of an angel here on earth.

In the beginning, I thought her age/size would play against her. But now, I believe it actually played a positive role in her ability to heal. To her body, this is all she knew and it seemed to respond so well because of that. Also, there is nothing as amazing as the child's mind. The ability to *worry* and create anxiety over her situation or condition did not exist. She has never complained about a thing, goes to the doctor as if it is what everyone does and is even willing to innocently donate her *baby* leg brace to her cousin, Baby Nicholas, because he is smaller than her and might need it (not realizing everyone doesn't wear a brace on their leg). She truly has played a huge part in her own personal healing. I can remember in the beginning of this all wondering, "Why me?" "What did I do wrong?"... Now, I'm still saying "Why me?" Except now, I can't imagine what I did right in life to deserve the blessing of Tori. She definitely has taught me more in her mere 4 years of life than I could ever learn in an entire lifetime on my own.

DAN WEIGAND
LUNG, LIVER & BONE CANCER

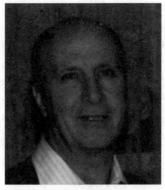

My journey began in December, 1999. I complained of lower back pain. The doctor could find no reason for it, so I was sent for x-rays. He ordered CT scans. I received the diagnosis in late January or early February 2000. I also had lab tests done at his office. The doctor advised IPT (Insulin potentiation therapy) as the main treatment.

Before staring the IPT, my prognosis was not good, even with IPT, so I researched to see if there was anything I could do to help myself. The first thing I did was get prayed for at church and get on prayer chains. I read a book I had by Jethro Kloss called *Back to Eden,* written in the 30s. He said disease can't live in pure blood, so I began to detoxify my body. Before I started treatment, I did a 10 day citrus juice fast, then I did carrot, parsley, and various greens. I drank pots of herb tea all day [red clover, milk thistle, golden seal, and dandelion].

At this time, I made major changes to my diet and lifestyle. I quit eating meat and sugar of any kind, drank steamed distilled water, and exercised.

Also, based on my lab tests, the doctor prescribed various supplements including aloe vera juice, enzymes, probiotics, pau d'arco tea, vitamins A&E, and D3. My treatment was once a week for ten weeks. It also included ozone therapy. There were no side effects from the treatment, which is about a 10 percent dose of chemotherapy. Halfway through the treatment, the doctor and I decided that I should go to the Midwest Cancer Treatment Center of America to try and determine the source of the cancer. I brought my tests and treatment history to have them review it. We met with an oncologist. He advised high-dose chemotherapy for my stage IV cancer, and said what I was currently doing was not a proper treatment. He also said the cancer could spread to my brain. I went through a battery of tests at that facility.

My wife was intimidated and scared by the doctor's demeanor, but I was comfortable with the treatment.

About two weeks later we received a call from the doctor at Midwest. He said he could not say I had cancer at that time, and that I should keep doing what I had been doing. This was Good Friday 2000. Needless to say, we had a joyfull Easter. I finished the balance of my treatments [4], and as of Jan. 2003, I am cancer free.

Some of the other books I read that helped me included *The Cancer Conqueror* by Greg Anderson, *How I Conquered Cancer Naturally* by Edie Mae, and *The Bible Cure* by Reginald Cherry, MD. Most important was learning to trust the Lord for my healing, because all good things come from above. Also, my doctor Ross Hauser of Caring Medical and Rehab Services, who has godly wisdom.

I believe the most effective part of my healing was staying with what I believed was God's direction for my treatment. Also, the comfort I received from his word, such as Psalm 103:1-3: "Praise the lord, o my soul; all my inmost being, praise his name. Praise the lord, o my soul, and forget not all his benefits — who forgives all your sins and heals all your diseases."

We must take responsibility for our own health and seek answers. I would like to add that my healing would not have occurred without the love and support of my wife, Sandy. She made the juices and teas and put up with my diet.

Twila J. Ritchie
Breast Cancer to the Bone

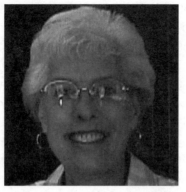

I requested a bone scan from my doctor after I started having muscle spasms in my lower back. I had been treated for breast cancer eight years earlier and had taken all the chemotherapy and radiation that the doctors recommended. I knew after the diagnosis that if I didn't find out what was behind this cancer, I would likely die. I had been in a Christian healing ministry for several years, so I turned to the Lord in prayer asking Him to show me what had happened in my life that had allowed cancer to occur.

In God's timing, I was shown that a spiritual death wish I had spoken into being fourteen years earlier had opened spiritual doors to darkness. I had said, "Is it going to take my dying for Jerry to wake up and see what is going on?" That statement is idolatrous. The base problem was a marriage that was on the rocks.

The doctor wanted me to have my bone marrow radiated, destroy my immune system and reinsert the bone marrow. There was only a 24% chance that it would work. I chose not to take this treatment. I felt led to go on a very healthy diet. Two books dropped in my lap, *Nutrition the Cancer Answer* by Maureen Sullivan and *The Cancer Battle Plan* by Ann Frahm. I followed them as best I could, as we had no organic health food stores where I live.

I also chose to take alternative treatment at the American Metabolic Institute. This treatment took place over a period of five weeks. I was told to get counseling for me and my husband when I returned home. The doctors knew how to get rid of the cancer, but they couldn't keep it from coming back. That has to come from within yourself. We did receive the necessary counseling which put our marriage on more stable ground. I continued on the diet for several months, as well as health supplements. At the end of a year and a half, a bone scan showed no cancer. A bone scan a year later was still clear.

There is no question in my mind that I would have died if I had not spoken the spiritual death wish out. The marriage also had to be healed of the more serious problems. God used the spiritual healing, diet and alternative treatments to bring about my healing from cancer.

CAROLE JAKABOSKI
INFLAMMATORY BREAST CANCER

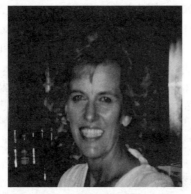

I was diagnosed in July of 2000. The cause of my cancer was the result of a near-fatal auto accident. I was forced off the road by a truck. My car went off the road and rolled down a cliff, turning over about 3 times. This accident caused mutation of cell in my left breast from the blunt trauma of injury to my chest and breast from the steering wheel. The cancer showed up seven and a half months later. I knew what it was the moment it appeared. It just blew up overnight with swelling, red, hot to touch, and very painful. I am a retired nurse, so, I didn't need anyone to tell me that I had the most dreaded of all types of breast cancer, with survival at the bottom of the scale. Of course, I was in shock, asking myself, "Why me?" I am a health nut, eat only the best organic food, lots of fresh fruits and veggies, and no smoking, drugs, or alcohol. Then I started to put two and two together and made the connection with the blunt trauma diagnosis.

I refused the horrible surgery that the American doctors had planned for me. My answer to their demand that I must have this done or I would die was, "You have given me one of two options: 1. Mutilation of my body and the loss of my chest and part of my arm and possible death from the trauma of the surgery and the anesthesia (I know I am allergic to the anesthesia) and death from the cancer when it spreads. Or, 2: Do nothing and die without the pain and suffering I would be inflected with from the surgery.

I did a lot of praying. The answer/miracle came to me from Dr. George who worked at the chiropractor's office. His friend had taken his mother to Dr. Donato Perez Garcia in Tijuana Mexico for IPT treatment. That stands for insulin potentiation therapy. Insulin is used as a magic bullet to carry the meds directly to the cancer cells, killing them and not killing the healthy normal cells. This gentle treatment has very few to no side effects. No hair loss, nausea, etc., as the standard chemotherapy that is given in the US does. From the first moment I laid eyes on Dr. Donato, I knew I was with the right doctor. I knew I was safe and that I would be treated by a real doctor, one who treats me as a whole human being, not just a cancer. I have never been treated with such love and kindness by any other doctor that I have seen. This man, Dr. Donato, is a true healer who says that he is doing what God has directed him to do for humanity.

I believe what healed me is the peace of mind from the loving treatment by Dr. Donato. The knowledge that I had new hope and the knowledge that I was an important human being, to this man, who has such respect for each and everyone of his patients.

TONY PRESTON
PANCREATIC CANCER

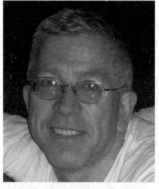

I was diagnosed with Pancreatic Cancer, Stage III, which became Stage IV within a month, with a tumor on a lymph node. In February 2001, my doctor told me to get my affairs in order. He said I would be disabled in 4 to 5 months and dead within 11 months. At about the same time, I found Protocel, and have been taking it since then. I did some chemotherapy, and my doctor said it had maybe a 20% chance of doing anything. In May 2001, my CA 19.9 was 4500 and has dropped steadily. Today, it is 100.

In March, I had a tumor on a lymph node in my groin area. First it got soft on the top, then the whole thing got soft and eventually it drained like a boil and then was completely gone. The drainage was sterile. Protocel is amazing stuff and has cured many people. The idea is that it lowers the energy production of all the cells in the body. Normal cells produce an excess and are not affected. Cancer cells barely produce enough energy to maintain themselves and will self-destruct. Pancreatic Cancer is one of the fastest killing cancers and there is very little that conventional medicine has to offer. Protocel is low cost, easy to take, and has been tested to be non-toxic. The original inventor, Jim Sheridan, wanted it to be available at a low cost, and it is.

Physically, I experienced the wasting away that many cancer patients have, for several months. I had fluid drained from my abdomen in January 2001, which is how I was diagnosed. My doctor told me I would have to be drained every couple of months, as the fluid is a side-effect of the cancer. I never needed to be drained again, since the fluid disappeared when the Protocel started to work. It took about 3 months before I started to physically gain weight. After that, I felt fine and continued to improve.

I have always had a strong faith in God, but when you are faced with cancer, your awareness in your mortality increases. I was not afraid of death, but was concerned for my family and what it would mean to them. I searched for help in various traditional sites like the National Cancer Institute (NCI) and found nothing. It was like a small miracle when I somehow (and to this day I cannot find the link that took me there) found information on Jim Sheridan and his treatment for Cancer.

Today, my doctor keeps telling me to *keep doing what you're doing*. It is a shame that a treatment like Protocel cannot be recommended to every cancer patient — it works. If it did not, I would not be here today.

I believe that God places the tools you need in your hands when you need them. I know that all the prayers of my family and friends were answered when I found the Protocel information.

I believe I was healed physically because Protocel worked a miracle. It stopped my cancer, it dissolved tumors, and prevented what was almost a certainty. Emotionally, the support from my wife and family was great, but even beyond that, I have had many acquaintances that, when they found out I had cancer, told me that they would be praying for me and adding me to their church's prayer list. It meant a lot to me, and I know that those prayers were being answered.

TERRY HERBERT
PROSTATE CANCER

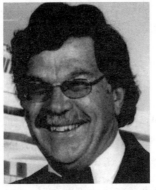

I was diagnosed in August 1996. I was 54 years old, which is said to be *young* for prostate cancer. The initial information that my wife, Anthea, and I were given was that my PSA was 7.2, my Gleason 3+3= 6 and I was staged T2bN0M0. We didn't know what this meant, but we knew I was going to die. And no one told us anything different.

Our reaction was shock, disbelief, anger, sorrow, and confusion. What to do? What will happen? It is difficult to put into words the tidal wave of feelings that swept over us, but from many discussions with people all over the world since then, it seems that our reaction was typical.

We really didn't know what to do. We had recently returned to South Africa after an absence of 15 years. We were about to start extensive alterations to the house we had bought. I was due to leave on a business trip to Australia within a fortnight. And now this! I am fairly phlegmatic, but Anthea has several Master's degrees in Worry and Concern, so she was really upset.

We started talking to everyone we knew to try and get a handle on the best way to deal with the problem. Someone suggested a visit to the Cancer Association. That thought hadn't even occurred to us! They were very empathetic and gave us copies of publications, which we found very helpful. An old friend of ours, a retired pediatrician, made some inquiries of his colleagues, and was the first person to tell us that not all prostate cancer is fatal. A business contact of mine, a man in his eighties who looks twenty years younger, pointed me in the direction of information on complementary and alternative medicine. And all these people were saying similar things — don't rush into surgery.

This was a surprise to us. The urologist had recommended Radical Prostatectomy and hadn't mentioned that there was more than one option for treatment. So we went back to him to ask him about these options and for a second opinion on the biopsy, having learned already that none of the tests used in diagnosis of prostate cancer is precise. It was only later that I learned that many of the tests he had ordered were also unnecessary, and very expensive!

He gave us more material. My biopsy came back with a lower Gleason Grade 2+3=5, which I now knew indicated a less aggressive tumor. I set off for my trip to Australia and Papua New Guinea, returning to South Africa through London. I had a stack of information and plenty of time to read on those long flights. By the time I got back home, I was pretty well convinced that surgery was not for me.

One of the books I had read was on the Bristol Centre in UK, which dealt with matters such as stress reduction, diet, meditation, visualization and exercise in the treatment of cancer. It made a lot of sense to us to try this approach, given the nature of prostate cancer progression and the fact that in the US, leading specialists acknowledge that most treatment of the disease is unnecessary. So we made the decision to start to change our lifestyle, our diet, and our habits. We did not do this with a huge lurch, but steadily; and it wasn't too difficult.

We continued with our research. I got onto the Internet and found a wealth of information there and a community of people from around the world who offered support and help. The more I read, the more it appeared to me that it might well be best for me not have any of the conventional treatments offered, but continue with the regimen I had started. Simplistically, my whole approach was, and still is, based on the premise that in normal circumstances the body's immune system and other mechanisms will deal adequately with cancer. Cells are mutating all the time, but very few of them develop and progress into tumors. The diagnosis of the cancer is an indicator that the system has failed, and it is therefore important to create an environment where the system can get back to do the work it is designed for.

The concept of visualization, which recurs in so much material dealing with complementary and alternative cancer therapies, appealed to me. I related my body and my cancer to an overgrown garden. Our house had such a garden when we bought it. It takes a good deal of hard work to rectify an overgrown garden, and a lot of time. Persistence is the name of the game. That is how I see my response to my disease. There is no doubt that the spontaneous remission of some cancers can take place in a very short time. There is a good deal of anecdotal material that tells of such regressions occurring overnight, and these are supported by a more limited number of medical testimonies. But because prostate cancer is a slow growing tumor, I never expected it to retreat any quicker than it grew.

It has not been easy following the path we have chosen. There is very little support for what is termed *Watchful Waiting* from friends and relatives and virtually none from the medical profession. I eventually found an oncologist who said he thought it might not be a bad idea, and a holistic doctor who helped in the early stages. But even subscribers to support and chat sites (on the Internet) still have some reservations and disagree with what I am doing. So it is a lonely path and, naturally, I ask myself often if it is wise to continue, especially when the odd ache or pain strikes. Things which one would normally take in one's stride as merely a function of growing a little older, or having exerted oneself too much, loom into my thoughts as, "Is this a spread?"

But apart from that, mentally and physically I am better than I have been for years. I cannot claim to be cured because there is no definition of cure for the path I have taken, and I am not sure that any doctor would even say that I was in remission. But I am in better health than I was when I was diagnosed, and there are no signs of progression of the disease. That's good enough for me.

A guest on an Oprah Winfrey show I saw years ago said that it was an unfortunate aspect of life that everyone needed a life-threatening experience to really appreciate how good life is. I agree with that! I believe prayer and faith in the Supreme Being and your body's ability to cure itself are enormously potent tools.

I don't think that there is any one thing which is more effective than others. The whole essence of wellness, to me, is the interaction of all we do and think — the wholeness of being.

I guess that one of the issues is my own attitude of mind. The late Stephen Jay Gould in his wonderful essay "The Median Is Not The Message" quotes Sir Peter Medawar, his personal scientific guru and a Nobelist in immunology, what the best prescription for success against cancer might be. "A sanguine personality," he replied.

Another quotation, which I keep in front of me at all times also seems appropriate. It is from *Flowers In Winter* by Sir William Keys and describes his doctor's reaction to his *cure* of prostate cancer by using Chinese medicines and meditation "… my personal observation, common to all *cures* has been the unshakable determination of the patient to show just how wrong (and usually how insensitive and apparently uncaring) those bloody doctors could be. The patients make up their minds to beat cancer and also to beat the doctor who implied they couldn't."

GARY SEIDEN
PROSTATE CANCER

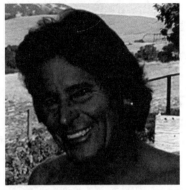

When I turned 50, I went in for a standard PSA test. I had been feeling fine, and with no symptoms that I was aware of. The score came in high, and I was totally shocked when after a biopsy, my doctor said I had an *advanced and aggressive* case of prostate cancer. His immediate recommendation was to have my testicles removed and my prostate radiated to slow the spread of the disease. My first question was, "How long do I have?" He said, "...Worst case one year, best case five years." I sought out two other opinions from leading doctors at both Stanford and UCSF Medical Center, and their estimates were the same.

This is the time that cancer patients remember most, and the time when patients are the most vulnerable to suggestions involving surgery, radiation or chemotherapy. We want to do anything to make it go away. But as we all come to know sooner or later, there is no magic pill. There is no one procedure that will *make it go away*.

I put off decisions regarding the surgery and radiation for about a month, and self-medicated with drugs and alcohol, contemplating my pending demise. But gradually, as I began to see through the haze, I started acquiring knowledge. I read about Western procedures, but more importantly about eastern, alternative and complementary therapies. I was unwilling to risk the side effects of surgery and radiation, and knew there had to be a better way. And this was the turning point — taking control of my own treatment decisions, rather than letting someone else do that for me. I realized that western doctors are for the most part interested in treating the symptoms, instead of the causes. A surgeon will suggest surgery. A radiologist, radiation. An oncologist, chemotherapy. Sometimes in the most extreme cases these procedures may be necessary and appropriate, but I knew the real answer was in myself, and in me being able to identify and follow my own path to a cure.

Based on my reading and gathering of information from many sources, I formulated a program based on diet, exercise, and attitude to strengthen my immune system so it would fight the cancer on its own, rather that relying on some external *cutting, burning or poisoning* that would further weaken the immune system. I came to believe that cancer is a systemic disease and not a local one, and as such should be treated accordingly.

And now, my life has never been better. I have become a more caring and compassionate person, and I treat every day as a gift. I spend time helping others, and this helps me in return. I try and be a role model for everyone else who is suffering from any kind of life threatening disease. And I have fun. I have taken up skydiving, mountain climbing, and travel as much as possible. I take long hikes and contemplate the beauty of nature and the spirit world. I am doing my best to give back at every opportunity.

The most effective part of my healing was making public my disease, and drawing on the love and support from friends and family to keep my spirits up. At first I kept it to myself. I was ashamed to admit I had cancer. Big mistake! Once I let it out, I got more and more love and support, and it made me stronger and determined not to let down all the people who were cheering me on.

The other most effective part was in gathering a team of

health care professionals. I have an herbalist, acupuncturist, massage therapist, chiropractor, and exercise training partners, as well as occasional visits to my western doctors. But it is the alternative and complementary therapies that I have the most faith in. They are the ones that keep my immune system healthy and fighting back the cancer.

JOE BROWN
MELANOMA CANCER

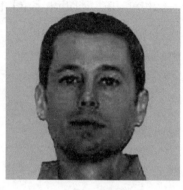

In 1997, a lymph node in the left side of my neck became badly swollen. I thought it was due to having a bad cold, and ignored it. Six months later, the lymph node was still severely swollen and I was coerced by my mother to have it checked out. I finally went to the doctor. The doctor ran tests for mononucleosis (mono), which came back negative. I was then sent to an ear/nose/throat doctor, who did a few needle biopsies. The biopsies indicated cell irregularities. An outpatient surgery was performed, and the swollen lymph node was removed and sent to pathology. Analysis confirmed cancer.

The diagnosis was late stage III melanoma in my neck lymph nodes and spreading. A second surgery was immediately scheduled and performed in which a few lymph nodes from the area of the swollen node were removed. Due to the rapid spreading and the known outcomes of late stage melanoma cancers, I was sent to see an oncologist. Dr. Issac, the oncologist, placed me on interferon alpha-2B, a drug that is supposed to stimulate the immune system. Interferons, which are a type of cytokines, are a class of immunotherapeutic drugs. I followed the strict regimen of the interferon for eight months. During the first month, I

received it intravenously, five days a week, at the doctor's
office. For the next seven months, I had to inject it into my
legs every other day three times a week. This treatment with
the interferon for the eight months cost over $150,000. The
medicine caused terribly severe muscle cramps, joint cramps
(especially in the knees and elbows) and occasional nausea.
I also felt *out of it* the whole time I was on this medicine. I
must admit, I have never felt physically worse ever in my
life. The cramps and joint pain were so severe a few times it
caused me to go into convulsions. As my mother frantically
dialed the doctors office and the emergency room trying
to get some information on what she could do, I honestly
thought I was going to die.

Every three months I was instructed to get CAT scans
and MRI's. When I was first placed on this interferon (after
the second surgery), the scans that were done showed no
cancerous cells in any of my lymph nodes. I know now that
even though these scans are sophisticated, they can only
pick up images of problems if the cells that are growing are
beyond a particular size. So while I took the interferon for
the eight months, thinking everything was okay, the small
cancerous cells that remained in some of the nearby lymph
nodes were rapidly growing and dividing. When they did a
second set of CAT scans and MRI's at the eighth month time
frame, the scans showed the cancer growing profusely and
that it had spread to many new lymph nodes.

At this point, my oncologist took me off the interferon,
seeing that it wasn't helping, and scheduled an immediate
surgery on Friday of that week. I was then informed that this
upcoming surgery was going to be all that could be done
surgically to try and stop the spread of the cancer. Also, that
one of the lymph nodes that was filled with cancer cells was
embedded in my sternocleidomastoid muscle in my left neck
region and that this muscle was going to have to be removed
as well. Dr. Simms, the ear/nose/throat doctor, who would
perform this radical neck section, told me that by the cutting
of this major muscle and damaging many of the nerves in

the localized region, that it was very possible that I would no longer be able to move my left arm. So now on top of the fact that mentally and physically I'm having to deal with cancer, which is draining in itself, trust me, now I was being told that there was a good chance that I would lose all mobility of my left arm, a shocking and unexpected blow.

After the surgery, I had an incision from behind my left earlobe down to my left clavicle and across my neck over under to my right earlobe. This was not a pretty sight, but somehow, by the grace of God, I could move my left arm. I was so thankful for this. After four long painful days in the hospital and a good month of healing and recuperating from this surgery, I had another appointment with my oncologist. During this meeting, he informed me that because the spread of my cancer was so fast and because the interferon didn't do what it was supposed to, he recommended I start high dose chemotherapy and radiation to stop the spread of any more cancer. He also told me that the chemotherapy was going to be a continuous drip, by IV, that would leave me in the hospital for at least a month, if not longer. With everything I had been through and with the light at the end of the tunnel not looking too bright at this point, he dropped the *bomb-shell* on me. He said, "At the rate your cancer is spreading, if you don't start the chemotherapy and radiation immediately, you will not survive the cancer." In other words, pack up your shit, because you just bought the farm.

It was at this point that my mother and I had some long talks about what could happen and started weighing the options. My mother remembered a long-time friend back east, a friend of my grandma, who had cancer many years back and who is still alive today. I spoke with him and he informed me of the Gerson diet and how he treated himself when he was dealing with his cancer. I also got on the Internet and started searching under alternative treatments, and by pure chance, I stumbled onto Dr. Daniel Rubin. Dr. Rubin is a naturopathic doctor who treats people by natural means, building up their immune systems so they can naturally heal themselves of their illness. At this point, I knew I had a bad feeling about the whole chemotherapy and radiation treatment. I didn't know much about it, but I did know that not only did the chemotherapy kill the bad cells, but it killed the good cells as well. And I knew if you are killing your good cells while being treated, this can't be such a good thing and it has to inhibit the whole process of your body fighting back and trying to rid itself of the disease. I made the decision to take my chances and to not do the chemotherapy and radiation.

In contrast to the oncologist, Dr. Rubin started by listening to me and finding out what had been going on. He offered only positive and reassuring advice and for the first time throughout this whole ordeal, I felt like my journey on this planet wasn't quite over. In the last surgery, twenty-three lymph nodes were removed from the left side of my neck and six nodes from the right side. The major gland that had been embedded within the muscle with a great number of the cancer cells within it, was kept at the hospital by the recommendation of Dr. Rubin. Now that I had made the decision to not do the chemotherapy and radiation, Dr. Rubin had that tumor sent to a clinic in Georgia. The facility in Georgia took the tumor antigens from the cancer and turned them into a tumor vaccine, called Dendritic T-cell stimulation (now being done at Aidan Inc., by Dr. Rubin). This series of shots (my tumor antigen, GM-CSF, and IL-2) was sent to me every month for the next six months. The idea of this vaccine is that it takes the tumor antigens from your tumor and by injecting them back into you causes your body to have a learned immune response to those specific cancer cells. This increases your body's immune system to have a specific response to any remaining cancer cells within the body. I injected the vaccine in the groin and stomach area using syringes. I also began treatments using alternative therapies, and went on a thorough detoxification program to detoxify the liver and clean out cancerous cells my body had already killed. I began receiving acupuncture treatments and

Dr. Rubin administered high dose Vitamin C IV's, which also contained all the B vitamins. He also started me on active hexose correlated compound (AHCC) and many vitamins and herbs. (AHCC is used in over 500 hospitals in Japan to treat cancer and AIDS.) Dr. Rubin networked with companies in Germany and acquired a powder, called Total Immune, which I took every day with water, that contained almost 200 vitamins and herbs at high potencies. On my own, I also took a variety of separate vitamin and mineral supplements including, zinc, colostrum, magnesium, calcium, burdock root, shiitake mushroom, garlic, aloe, and pau d' arco. I consumed pau d' arco in tablet form and also drank pau d' arco tea. I bought aloe vera juice and drank it. I bought fresh garlic from the store, peeled it, and would eat three to five cloves a day. At night I would drink a mouthful of apple cider vinegar. I also drank Essiac tea and green tea.

I strictly followed the Gerson diet, which I researched extensively. Three times a day I juiced two Granny Smith apples and six carrots and immediately drank the fresh juice. I would sometimes add things like oranges or beets for variety and to help clean the liver. The most important part of the Gerson diet is to intake no salt, no refined sugar, no wheat, no dairy products, no meat, and no canned vegetables, which I held to exclusively. I ate salmon regularly because of the high levels of omega-3, -6, -9 fatty acids. So my diet mainly consisted of juices, salads, fruits, vegetables, and salmon.

I was also fortunate enough to be going through this when Dr. Shakar from India was teaching at the Southwest College Medical Center. Dr. Shakar is extremely knowledgeable with cell salts, which he prescribed me. I also went through mind/body therapy, in which I visualized different methods of myself killing the cancer. I strongly believe that the mind plays a big part in illnesses a person gets and how you can aid your body to get rid of them.

Nothing Dr. Rubin gave me caused side effects and the cost of my natural treatment with Dr. Rubin didn't even put a dent in the money it cost for the interferon alpha-2B drug that I was administered by my previous oncologists. I did better both physically and mentally with this natural approach the whole time I was on it then I did in one week with my previous oncologist (I'll let you pick the week.).

I continued to see the ear/nose/throat doctor, who kept track of the cancer through CAT scans and MRI's. After the treatments with Dr. Rubin, I not only felt better, but I knew I was going to be better. Every month I submitted my blood work to be tested at the clinic in Georgia. I was able to track the increase in my T-cells, CD-8's, and Natural Killer cells. Not only was I feeling better with more energy, but I could watch my progress on paper every month. Within the first few months, my white blood cells more than doubled the amount that I had when I first started treatment.

It is now June of 2002. I still have MRI's about every six months to a year, and they still show me to be cancer free. I went from a situation where the oncologists offered me no hope to a situation where I met some naturopathic doctors who not only gave me hope, but gave me a treatment that would cure me. These naturopathic doctors also treated my whole condition for a fraction of the cost that the interferon alpha-2B cost alone (not to mention all the CAT scans, MRI's, X-rays, etc.). I believe so much in the philosophy of natural medicine and the belief that if you give your body what it needs it will rid itself of any and all illnesses, that I am now enrolled in Southwest College of Naturopathic Medicine. I took my college degree from A.S.U. and applied to only one medical school — this one. I want to learn everything Dr. Rubin and the other doctors who treated me knew when they offered me hope when everyone else shut the door on me. I am about to start my second year here at Southwest College of Naturopathic Medicine and plan on entering the medical field and working with cancer patients.

They say in life things happen for a reason, that you might not always understand that reason, but that there is one. I believe this. I now positively know that my higher positioning on this earth is to help other people with cancer, by using the latest medical experience combined with alternative therapies. I plan on helping and curing people to the best of my ability. I will help and cure people. It is now going on 5 years, and I am healthy and happy, and I am still cancer free.

I honestly believe the most effective part of my healing was meeting Dr. Daniel Rubin, N.D. This man did more for me than any other in terms of curing me. I honestly feel if it weren't for the Dendritic T-cell stimulation, the AHCC, the juicing, the different combinations of vitamins and herbs, I wouldn't be here today. I believe so much in this medicine that I plan on helping and teaching others as I have been helped.

DR. GEORGE HADLEY
PROSTATE CANCER

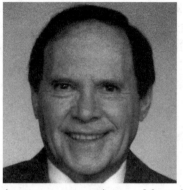

I used to be a kidneystone producer. My original diagnosis came about through a routine visit to my urologist. When he mentioned the big *"C"* I was stunned. Other than the stones, I had lived a healthy life. I was raised by a registered nurse and she had taught me to take care of myself and to stay as clear of doctors as I could. I am 70, and except for the urologist visits for the kidneystones, I have only seen a doctor maybe ten or so times in my life. The doctor that diagnosed me had a very negative attitude and scared me big time, so I fired him and decided to handle this thing on my own.

My wife and I have our own business, so she kindly gave me whatever time I needed to cure myself, shouldering the burden of the business herself. I am eternally grateful to her for that. I immediately read everything on health and curing cancer I could, and set about building a regimen for myself. I am a very disciplined person, so it was easy for me to follow the routine I developed. Since we make our living writing, I put it all into a book titled, *The Wellness Book*. It is not just about curing cancer or any other serious health problem; it is really about living a healthy life physically, emotionally, and spiritually.

Basically I did the following five things:

1. Supplements: I use Usana products. After looking at many, I found they seem to have the best research and development behind them. (I have sold enough friends on using them that I get a check each month that more than covers what I use — Neat.)

2. Diet: I changed my way of eating. I cut way back on sugars (that was tough) and unhealthy fats and adding more raw fruits and vegetables. I found several healthy dips that made the raw veggies easier to take. I still ate fish and chicken in moderation, but cut out most other meats.

3. Fasting and Colonics: I read several good accounts of how important it is to clean out the intestines so I wasn't poisoning myself. I started out by fasting eight days, only drinking juice. I did two coffee colonics a day. What I cleaned out of my intestines you don't want to hear. I also took cleansers Sonne #7 and #9 available at health stores to clean out the small or upper intestines. Once the colon is clean the nutrients can get into the bloodstream.

After the eight day fast, I would fast and do colonics once a week to stay clean. I continue to do the eight day fast twice a year and fast one day a week the rest of the time.

4. Exercise: I began exercising three times a week. I did a mile or more of walking at a brisk pace and half hour on the body machines toning my upper and lower body. I was beginning to slouch over before that, but soon was standing up straight again and looking good.

5. Meditation and Prayer: I meditated and prayed 20 minutes a day. It was during one of these meditations that my pain went away. After my diagnosis, I began to manifest the usual prostate symptoms. One of them was pain down my right leg and in my side and groin. It got so bad one day that I went to bed to meditate and pray that God take this pain away. I was really praying in earnest because it hurt bad and finally I screamed, "God, take this pain away NOW!!!! I don't want it. I don't need it. Take it away NOW!!!"

And in less than fifteen minutes the pain went slowly away and has never come back. I believe in prayer, but that was a miracle. Of course, I thanked God profusely.

I have had no signs of the cancer since taking the time to heal, and at 70, I am in as good a shape as when I was in my 30s and 40s. I hike five miles per week, mostly up and down mountains around San Diego. I plan on living to be 120 or more. My mom is 93, works full time with *old people* and is going strong. She even has a new boyfriend.

My wife Lynéa is a healer. Following what she teaches, setting goals, discovering and eliminating any blocks to those goals, and most importantly not giving in to fear and worry, I believe have accounted for my health success. She teaches that what you see and focus on in your mind becomes your life. If you focus on fear and worry, you get more to fear and worry about. But if you see yourself as healthy and healed and truly believe it is so, a *done deal* as she says, then that is what you get. Setting definite goals and following through is the disciplined part of health and healing. Seeing yourself as healthy and healed is the mind work, equally important, in fact, the basis for everything else you do. Seeing myself as healed and believing it was so, I feel, was the key to my healing.

ROBIN RESSEL
BRAIN STEM GLIOMA

Miracles happen to people every day and there's no reason why one can't happen for us. This was the philosophy I adopted when my eleven-year-old daughter, Jessica was diagnosed with cancer. That word has to be the most frightening in the English language. When you're told your child has a terminal illness that there is no cure for, it feels like a sharp needle piercing the center of your heart. The pain is so intense and unbearable it's hard to describe in words the physical impact you feel. It's like a blow to the head, you don't see coming, then pow! You're knocked flat on your back. Looking back, I can see why the doctor acted so nervous and looked so pale when he asked my husband and me to wait in his office. When he shared the news with us, we were devastated without an ounce of hope. Maybe this is why some people just give up and often times accept the inevitable. It's so sad to hear when someone turned to a conventional cancer treatment especially knowing the brutality to their quality of life.

In March 1996, Jessi was diagnosed a brain stem glioma. Severely crossed eyes were the only symptom she had. In only two weeks her eyes went from looking really bad to horrible. Anything beyond eighteen inches would double. Her tumor was an astrocytoma and it was impossible to know the stage since no biopsy could be done. She had a pea size monster sitting deep in the middle of her head waiting to take her life. The only option offered to us was standard radiation. Of course we asked about the gamma knife and other specialty types of radiation as well as chemo, but in Jessi's case there just simply was nothing else. Thank God for a very honest doctor. We were told chemo wouldn't penetrate the blood brain barrier and informed about the cruel side effects of what radiation does to a person's body. It may be an option if you're zapping a spot on an arm or leg but inside the center a young persons head, there is was no way we would ever dream of putting our daughter through that! Jessi's life expectancy was anywhere from eight to eighteen months with or without treatment. We also were informed that radiation will often times add fuel to the fire, cause a tumor to grow faster, and could take her life even sooner. Once our doctor shared this harsh evil reality with us we knew we had to find an alternative.

After a lot of prayers and endless searching I found Dr. S. R. Burzynski in Houston, Texas. The antineoplaston therapy he discovered is non-toxic medicine that virtually has no side effects. I can't even begin to tell the number of times I have heard of a conventional medical doctor slam Dr. Burzynski with every comment from quack to snake oil. I have been asked many times if this medicine is really a cure for cancer and so wonderful, then why doesn't everyone know about it. Unfortunately there is no one easy answer. My usual answer is because of politics, power and money. A book called *The Burzynski Breakthrough* by Tom Elias and the web address www.burzynskipatientgroup.org are a couple excellent resources to know more history.

When Jessi was diagnosed, the very first thing I did was read and research everything about brain tumors and nutrition that I could get my hands on. I discovered that Antineoplastons is gene therapy. This is the only type of medicine I know of that has anti-cancerous properties. The medicine acts like a set of instructions to telling your cells how to grow. When a cancerous cell dies then a healthy one grows in its place. Dr. B. has treated his patients with excellent success since 1977.

The clinic was operating just fine until about 1983 when the federal government began to cause problems and put their big foot in the door. Part of the FDA was literally trying to shut the clinic down when another part of the FDA approved Dr. B. to go ahead with phase II clinical trials. When Jessi was diagnosed, my family and I had no choice but to become politically active and joined the rest of the

Burzynski supporters to fight for patients rights.

In the fall of 1996, we went to Washington DC with about 70 Burzynski supporters. Earlier in June of that same year, while on one of Jessi's doctor visits, we attended a democratic party fund raiser where Bill Clinton spoke in downtown Houston. Fourteen Burzynski supporters also attended. The message we were trying to get across was that the patient (not the government) has the right to choose their own medicine and doctor. The Burzynski Clinic still continues to operate under phase II clinical trails. The worst part was that we were more worried about Jessi losing the access to her life-saving medicine than we were about her cancer.

In May 1997 Jessi and I, along with little brother Kevin, who was only four months old, went to Dr. B's second trial in Houston. Just like the first trail held in January, this trial was also a big farce. It ended in a not guilty verdict and the clinic still continued to carry on treating patients.

Jessi is now eighteen and a high school senior. She runs cross country and track. She has a part-time job and goal of saving for her own car. She has reached the point where her social life is more important, and heaven forbid she actually has to spend time with her parents. Parents are now considered geeks unless, of course, she wants to borrow money or the car. Her last MRI was in October 2002 and showed no trace of cancer. We'll soon reach the five year mark of Jessi's remission and she'll only need an MRI every other year. Our other two kids are Willy, age fourteen, and Kevin, age six. Willy is at the "just don't talk to me in public or in front of anyone" phase. He plays the tuba and is the major athlete of the family. At the present time, he keeps us the busiest. Soon, little brother will follow in his footsteps and keep us even busier. All kidding aside, the other two aren't so bad just at completely different stages than Kevin. Kevin is a nice little ego boost. He still thinks mom and daddy are wonderful. I know that will change soon enough.

Several people have shared with me how unbelievably

strong I was all through Jessi's illness. When you know losing your child's life is not an option, the only thing you can do is pray for all the courage and strength the good Lord can send you. In our case, the Lord also blessed us with a bonus when I became pregnant with Kevin. I guess it was the God's way to let us know everything would be all right and to help us focus on something more positive. It has been said "God will only give us what we can handle." That was one challenging year and I'm glad it is over. When I think of a cancelled flight in a busy airport, with a fussy baby, and a whining kid on a cancer treatment... Honestly, the only way I got through each day was by God's pure grace! To have a healthy teenager even though she can drive us all crazy at times is certainly a miracle and worth it!

TORREY MORSE
LYMPHOMA

Not many people believe me when they learn that I have had cancer. I am 33, a new home owner and a workaholic, who has always been involved in a variety of extracurricular activities, from varsity volleyball in high school to hiking, to oversea travel during college and since. Today, baking cakes for sale, taking salsa dance lessons and enjoying mountain biking help fill my time away from the office. I have a Masters in Education and am a Certified Vocational Rehabilitation Counselor. Most people with whom I come in contact are unaware that I am also a cancer survivor. Twenty-five years this year!

October 9, 1978 I was diagnosed with Diffuse Histiocytic Lymphoma an aggressive Non-Hodgkin's Lymphoma, uncommon in children. I was 8 years old and had undergone a routine tonsillectomy. Within a week's time I experienced the rapid growth of a tumor in the place of my left tonsil. Upon removal of the tumor I began chemotherapy at Yale New Haven Hospital in New Haven, Connecticut. My parents were told that with a two to three year regimen of chemotherapy and possible cranial radiation my prognosis would be five to seven years. After three months of chemotherapy I was not doing very well. At that time there was little variance between treatment dosages of chemotherapy for children and adults. I became bloated and lost my hair. I often vomited within the first hour after receiving my outpatient treatments. The vomiting would usually continue for several hours and throughout the night. Chemotherapy was halted when I became exposed to the flu and then Chicken Pox. The doctors informed my parents that since my white cell count was low and my immune system weak, I would likely have a severe case of the Chicken Pox. Although I was given an injection of Gamma Globulin to diminish this possibility and stayed with a family friend while my sister, Jessica, was ill, they were correct.

During that time in February 1979, my parents made a decision to explore other cancer treatment options. They read about Laetrile available in Mexico, a Vitamin C therapy offered by Dr. Linus Pauling, and they researched a variety of nutritional approaches such as a Macrobiotic Diet. Through a friend in our church they learned about Dr. John T. Beaty in Greenwich, Connecticut who shared with them information about a new non-toxic therapy, Immuno-Augmentative Therapy (IAT), which treats an individual's immune system. He informed my parents that IAT was researched and offered at a clinic in the Bahamas by founder Dr. Lawrence Burton. Lawrence Burton Ph.D had begun his cancer research at New York University in 1955, and prior to opening the IAT Clinic had spent 11 years at St.Vincent's Hospital in Long Island, New York where as a Senior Investigator and Zoologist his research had focused on the factors involved in cancerous tumor growth and the blood components of the human body's immune defense system.

On March 16, 1979, my mother and I flew to Freeport, Grand Bahama Island, Bahamas so that I could begin treatment at the Immuno-Augmentative Research Centre. Dr. Beaty had strongly recommended Dr. Burton's treatment and advocated for Dr. Burton to accept me as his first child patient. He had seen Dr. Burton's success first hand in his nurse, Becky Hall who was treated for Esophageal Cancer. Becky's esophagus had been burned by radiation treatment and she had nearly died. She went to the IAT Centre for further treatment. Dr. Beatty told my parents that Dr. Burton's therapy, which was comprised of immuno-protein injections did not cause debilitating side effects such as those often associated with orthodox cancer treatments. In fact he stated that there were no side effects other than occasional fatigue. My parents opted for pursuing a treatment, which would allow me a better quality of life. Their decision I believe has played a significant role in my being alive today.

The IAT treatment is not what orthodox medicine would

classify as an aggressive treatment, but is an individualized treatment that works with one's immune system aiding it to fight the cancer. It doesn't work overnight; it takes time. Thus, a new patients' initial time was 6-8 weeks when I started in 1979 and today it is 8-12 weeks. Each patient receives a daily blood pull to monitor the immune system and to determine the best combination of sera, serum injections, needed. The blood test developed by Dr. Burton evaluates the relative activity of the body's natural tumor kill process and immune responses. Injections of sera are prescribed by timing and sequence to promote immunologic response. (IAT Pamphlet, 2000) Currently, patients return every four months for a two-week *tune-up* following their initial visit. In between visits the clinic provides each individual with serum and a printout to prepare a series of daily injections just as he or she has while at the clinic. This routine continues until the individual is told otherwise. The next step: return visits every six months for two weeks, and for some, eventually once a year.

My mother and I stayed in Freeport for six weeks initially. I then returned to the island every six months for a five day *tune-up*. Following each visit to the island, I was provided with serum and a six-month schedule of injections, for my *maintenance treatment*. Every six weeks I would visit Dr. Beatty and have a blood pull that would be sent to the IAT Centre in the Bahamas. My injection schedule was adjusted as necessary. During my third visit to the clinic in November 1980 Dr. Burton informed my mother and me that I would no longer need to receive treatment except when at the clinic for *tune-ups*. One year later, after just two days at the clinic for my fifth visit, Dr. Burton said to go home and spend the Thanksgiving day holiday with my family. In addition, I did not need to return for a year. I have since continued to return to the clinic annually for the most part. As an adult I have never been away from the IAT clinic for more than a two-year period. Although I could probably stay away longer, an annual *tune up* in the Bahamas has simply become a part of my life.

The following is an excerpt of a paper I wrote as a sixth grader regarding my experience with cancer. It was the fall of 1980 just prior to what would be my third *tune-up* visit at the IAT Centre. I was eleven years old.

It has been a terrible experience for my family and me during these two years I have had cancer. The beginning fears, treatment, decisions that were made, and traveling in and out of the country. However, I know I will be fine and that, because my parents love me and trusted God, they were able to get through and make hard choices. My family has come closer to each other, and believes God has used Dr. Burton as a tool in healing me. I was fortunate that my family found, and felt they had the right to make a choice of, treatment for me. I believe they made the right choice. (Morse, 1980)

Twenty-two and half years later my opinion has not changed. It is my faith in a higher power and belief in the right as an individual to make choices about my personal wellness and healthcare that I share with others. And of course, information about a very special cancer clinic located in the Bahamas.

Immuno-Augmentative Therapy (IAT) is an individualized treatment. In the twenty-six years since its founding in 1977, the IAT Centre has treated over 5,000 people who have had a wide variety of cancers, and many, surely a greater percentage than would likely have in this country, have lived longer healthier lives. However, not everyone responds as well as I have. Type/grade of cancer, age, stage, immune system function prior to onset of illness, lifestyle (diet, exercise, smoking, drugs, etc), how long one has been battling cancer and previous treatment affects/complications play a role in the success.

I know many people with diagnoses of colon, liver, breast, malignant melanoma, lymphoma and other cancers, who are alive and well, 5,10,17, 20 and 25 years later. Most of these people still return to IAT on a yearly basis or more frequently. Sometimes those visits become a family affair. I now have two aunts who have been to the clinic. One is a 12-year survivor of Pseudomyxoma Peridtnei, a rare abdominal cancer. The other is just completing her second year in treatment for Uterine cancer. Several individuals, who like me, have gone off the serum other than when at the clinic, have experienced reoccurrence, and have gone back on the injections full time. Others I have met responded well to the treatment, but did not get to the IAT clinic soon enough. Letters of gratitude, however, sent to the clinic from family members and friends voicing thankfulness for the additional time and quality of life their loved ones gained, and numerous survivor stories like my own, are evidence of Dr. Burton's achievement.

A pioneer in unorthodox cancer research, Dr. Burton passed away in May of 1993. The IAT Centre continues to survive under the direction of Dr. R. John Clement, who has been involved since its inception. Three medical doctors are available to address the daily medical concerns of patients, and offer weekly planned or ad hoc discussions on a variety of wellness related topics. Staff do their best to assist patients with all their needs, from living arrangements and car rentals to planning annual Thanksgiving and Christmas Dinners. For many patients, myself included, the IAT Centre is a home away from home, in part due to tenured staff who are not just employed, but who are dedicated to maintaining the existence of a therapy they have seen work. Dr. Clement and the IAT staff make no unkept promises, but practice a motto of honesty as they educate prospective patients about what IAT has to offer, and continually inform current patients of treatment status and likely prognosis.

Other publications, which offer information about the IAT Clinic and other alternative cancer therapies include *New Cancer Therapies: The Patient's* by Penelope Williams (Canada: Firefly Books, 2000) and *Cancer Syndrome 'Proven Methods'* (New York: Grove Press Books, 1980) and other titles by Ralph Moss.

My personal story and the journey my family experienced in choosing to pursue an alternative cancer therapy is told from my mother's perspective in *Torrey's Miracle - A Matter of Choice* (1st Books Library, 2001) and can be obtained via the Internet at www.1stbooks.com or directly from her.

Both my mother, Margaret Berger Morse, and I can be contacted via email at cplottie@aol.com.

ANN FONFA
BREAST CANCER

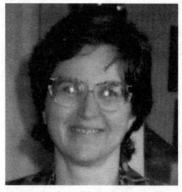

I had a lumpectomy and axillary dissection (18 negative nodes, which were removed without my express consent). I refused radiation, as a paper had just been published showing overall survival was the same for lumpectomy alone, versus lumpectomy with radiation, versus mastectomy with tumors under 2 cms.

I also refused chemo, as studies showed it was not very effective with slow-growing cancer cells and Stage 1 disease. Plus, I was very chemically sensitive (quite a bit better now) and the oncologist simply dismissed it.

I wanted the treatment to be more personalized than it seemed. I had been a vegetarian for the 18 years prior to diagnosis and made some adjustments to my diet, for example, giving up cheese, and changing type of fat (adding flax oil and more Omega 3).

Two years later I found another lump and I had a second lumpectomy, which found that lump to be malignant and another under it as well. (The second one did not show up on the mammo or sono-gram). Again I refused radiation. This time the growth rate of the cancer cells had slowed to less than normal cells and two oncologists told me NOT to do chemo.

I began Metabolic Enzyme Therapy (with Dr. Jack Taylor) and used lots of digestive enzymes. I also had colonics and began coffee enemas daily. Although I saw benefits with this program, I continued to develop more tumors.

My (second) surgeon told me that since I had 'multi-focal' disease, it was not really a recurrence, but rather a slow-developing cancer in most of the breast tissue.

After a third lumpectomy, I traveled to Canada to meet Gaston Naessons and try 714X. I used one cycle of the drug, but needed another biopsy as I developed 6 new tumors around my nipple.

I finally agreed to a mastectomy, as it seemed every inch of the breast tissue was indeed malignant. I refused the chest wall radiation offered.

I decided to travel to Mexico and try the Gerson Therapy at CHIPSA (then run by the Gerson Research Organization). I was there for two weeks accompanied by my mother. I was probably the healthiest person ever to go there. Although I had multiple tumors develop, the disease had never gone beyond local recurrences.

When I returned home, I kept up the Gerson program for the full eighteen months. It was not easy, but I got into a rhythm and schedule for all the activities needed.

However, while on this therapy I developed a tumor on the chest wall (still in local breast tissue). I decided to use 'high-dose' vitamin A therapy. I also increased the other basic anti-oxidants, E, C and selenium as a balance. The program I chose to follow combined elements I had heard about from several sources. It included 300,000 IU of Vitamin A daily for the first week. Then 150,000 daily for the next 4 weeks, then 2 weeks off. I added 2400 IU Vitamin E and about 12 grams of C (as ascorbic acid) with 400 mcg of selenium.

After just three weeks, I saw a reduction in the tiny tumor on my chest wall. However, when I tried to show it to the oncologist I used for blood work, he failed to look, measure, photograph or otherwise pay attention to it.

I continued the 'high-dose' protocol for about 14 months.

I then had the tumor surgically removed. Results: very few malignant cells, very well differentiated and the ER and PR receptor status had tripled. All excellent results.

However, a new tiny tumor had been developing during the last few months which clearly was not responding to the protocol. I began using Maitake Mushroom Extract (D-fraction) as I knew the company had begun clinical trials here in the U.S. This worked to reduce the tumor.

Later I developed more and had them surgically removed. My surgeon suggested there was not much more breast tissue and the 'next' surgery might require a plastic surgeon to be involved.

I was determined not to use any more surgery.

Yet one year later, my right breast developed Paget's Disease of the Nipple. Since the one thing all the doctors had told me about invasive lobular (my original diagnosis) was that it often spread to the second breast, I was persuaded this had happened.

I asked for a mastectomy — I just could not face much more surgery. However, I refused axillary dissection as this time I had a choice. I asked the surgeon to 'slice and dice' the breast and have pathology tell us what was going on inside of it.

She informed me that they found NO tumor and it was being called a Stage 0. She also said 'we' made the right decision not to do the axillary dissection.

I was emotionally devastated by the loss of my second breast. For some reason that seemed worse to me than other problems I had encountered. I am a very sexual woman and I loved my breasts. I first 'developed' at age 10 1/2 and was quite satisfied with the life I had with them.

Now I wondered to myself if I was 'still a woman'? I agonized and tormented myself and friends and family. My partner told me many times that I was more important than my breasts.

I knew that, but could not accept it. It took about ten months to settle down. I was happy to read a study that suggested that developing a Stage 0 disease was a sign that the body was fighting back.

Over the years I had read so much, gathered so much information, I started a group in 1994 to discuss CAM. I handed out packets of information at breast cancer meetings, I spoke to groups, including Cancer Care, Inc.

In 1997 I began The Annie Appleseed Project designed to inform and educate the public on issues of CAM. In June, 1999 we put up a website. The protocol I use and all of the issues around it are shown on our website site under *Ann's Bio* at www.annieappleseedproject.org.

I have been MRI-proven *No Discernible Disease* for about the last three years. I credit the Chinese herbs I take.

GAYLE CRANFORD
BREAST CANCER

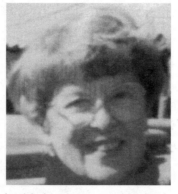

I was diagnosed with breast cancer. In August of 1984, I began chemo, but stopped in December after reading material about alternative treatments.

When I quit chemo that December, I began a metabolic treatment with an MD northwest of Pittsburgh.

I changed my diet to vegetarian, juiced and detoxed daily, and used many supplements.

In 1986 I flew to San Diego and integrated the program from the Livingston Foundation Medical Clinic there. The program, using some injectables and similar supplements already being used, included a vaccine. I continue to visit the clinic every other year now.

I began to feel better than I had in a long time.

Emotionally, I have felt empowered taking charge of my own illness and making decisions that didn't always agree with my doctors.

I sometimes think that God must have known that I would be interested enough to become very involved in spreading the word and helping others. I have tried to give direction to over 300 cancer patients over the years.

I believe I was healed by diet change and detoxification.

SUE VANDERWATER

MELANOMA

At the age of 25 I went for a routine visit to my doctor for a PAP smear and other routine examination procedures. I just happened to mention to him that I had a very black mole just under the right rib cage that seemed to be growing so quickly that I could virtually watch it! He was very quick to suggest a biopsy. Two weeks went by with no word from the clinic, and so I thought all was well. However, the fateful call finally came at work one day just a week before Christmas in 1977. My doctor approached the subject by asking me, "Who's your favorite surgeon?" He proceeded to tell me that the diagnosis was malignant melanoma and I could wait until after Christmas to have a wide excision of the area if I wanted to. However, what little I knew of cancer at that time was that once it had been released into the blood stream, it would travel to other parts of the body and set up house.

I insisted that he perform the surgery right away, before Christmas. When the surgeons were finished taking 5 inches in diameter and 7 layers of skin, I vowed that I would never be pressured into this type of surgery again and would find out the cause of this disease, if possible.

As I studied, it became obvious to me that I had exposed myself to numerous toxins, the most deadly being a paint stripper with which I was working. A poor diet, composed largely of Pepsi and nutritionless foods, was certainly a component as well, in my opinion. And so I set about researching the solution to this illness.

While attending a Chiropractic convention in Las Vegas, I discovered a book called *Cancer Winner* by Jacquie Davison that detailed her battle with malignant melanoma. The chosen therapy was Dr. Max Gerson's work, a therapy which rebuilt the immune system while detoxing the body. I absorbed all the information in the book and began collecting an entire library on the subject including Dr. Gerson's book

Cancer Therapy: Results of 50 Cases.

When I returned home to Michigan, I set up a very organized methodology of implementing the therapy on a daily basis and began finding various doctors of alternative medicine to help me monitor the results of the therapy and supply the supplements that were required. I remained on the therapy for approximately 3 years.

Twenty-four years have gone by, but in many ways my life has been changed forever. Many components of the therapy became a way of life, such as the distilled water, consciousness of toxins in the environment, eating *live* foods rather than *dead* ones, and much, much more.

You can't go back.

The juicing and coffee enemas definitely were rebuilding and detoxing at the same time. A "Type A" personality that will not give up during the implementation of the therapy is definitely key to my healing as well.

Elizabeth Vought
Breast Cancer

I never thought I would get breast cancer since we have no cancer in our family history. Also, I have taken care of myself for many years, being a vegetarian for 30 years and working out at the gym 4 times a week for the last 20 years.

In June 1999, I was injured while being shown a martial arts move by a friend, who fell on my upper right breast exactly where a 6 cm lump arose all at once within two months. As this accident happened, I was thinking to myself that this could cause breast cancer, since my mother had warned me at a young age to be careful of being hit in the breast because it could cause breast cancer. Within seconds, immediately after the accident, my friend said, "Oh no, breast cancer," I was surprised he had also heard the same thing. I had decided that it was an old wives tale and examined the area weekly after the accident, as well as giving myself examinations in the past on a monthly basis. I know I was okay before the accident.

Within six weeks, or so, I noticed that the whole area that was injured started elevating into a smooth, flat, disk shaped, moveable lump. I looked for swollen lymph nodes under my arm and finally found one in August of 1999, two months after the accident.

I immediately went to a reputable breast clinic in Santa Monica, California, called Joyce Kiefer Eisenberg Breast Center at St. John's Hospital to have a mammogram. After the mammogram, I met with the radiologist. He had compared my previous baseline mammogram taken 8 years earlier with the new mammogram, and he said he saw no change and did not see anything suspicious. He told me that I was fine and to "go home and forget about it." I asked him why I had a swollen lymph node which showed up on the mammogram, and he said, "I don't know; sometimes women get them and they never go down." I went home relieved, thinking that the lump was a fat necrosis from the accident. However, ten months later I decided to make an appointment with a different doctor, since the skin above the lump started taking on a bruised look after taking a hot shower one night.

The new doctor was alarmed, so I decided to have a biopsy immediately and found that it was malignant. I realized at that point that mammograms do not work on me, and I was surprised that the radiologist did not suggest an ultrasound 10 months earlier. I had not realized that mammograms do not work 25 to 30 percent of the time. My doctor felt that in order to have a successful lumpectomy, I should shrink the lump first by taking 4 treatments of Adriamycin-cytoxin and 4 treatments of Taxol, all three weeks apart, so I did. I was frightened and decided to do this treatment, since my doctor also told me that nothing else worked.

For six months I went through a very uncomfortable chemo treatment, losing my hair, periods, etc. I noticed that most of the women taking chemo were back for the second and third time because the cancer had spread deeper after previous chemo treatments and surgery. This felt wrong and frightened me into researching alternative treatments. I had heard about the Ralph Moss Report (website: cancerdecisions.com) and decided to order a report for my type of cancer. This is where I learned of Dr. Bicher's clinic, Valley Cancer Institute. Mr. Moss spoke highly of Dr. Bicher's treatment, so I immediately made an appointment with Dr. Bicher and decided to start treatment 2 weeks after my last chemo treatment, starting in the middle of December of 2000. (When I started treatment at Valley Cancer Institute, my tumor had reduced from chemo to about 4.5 cm and I had six swollen lymph nodes under my arm the size of marbles).

At Valley Cancer Institute, I went through approximately six months of low-dose radiation and hyperthermia, 5 days a week, taking about 2 hours a day. The treatment was easy, relaxing and painless. I read and slept through all of the treatments and afterwards went about my day normally.

Today, I am cancer free. I have all my lymph nodes that have gone back to their normal size, and my breast is normal. My MRI and tumor markers are normal. All I can say is it was a real learning experience and I'm glad I made it, thanks to Dr. Bicher and his people at Valley Cancer Institute. I sincerely feel that the treatment works very well. I also feel more enlightened after going through the cancer experience. It can give a person a better outlook on life. I feel more appreciative about my life. I've met some good friends through this experience, and overall look at life differently, in a more positive way. In other words, good things can come out of bad things.

I also truly believe that accidents can trigger cancer. I researched UCLA medical library and there are many articles on the subject, although the library does not keep copies of these articles for some reason. After the research I have done, I believe that we all have cancer cells that our immune system controls or they stay inactive until a trauma happens that injures the surrounding tissue, leaving the cancerous cells activated to multiply. I have met many people during my cancer treatment that had the same type of experience I did. I suggest that if you are hit hard to watch it closely.

I feel that the hyperthermia and low-dose radiation was the most effective part of my treatment. Since I already took care of myself, I knew I needed to target the cancer through some type of treatment and hyperthermia and low-dose radiation made sense to me. I think eating healthy food is important, staying away from sugar and dairy is a good idea. Also I did a lot of praying for guidance to find a treatment that would work to get rid of the cancer, and God answered my prayers.

Vernon Jones
Neck Cancer

On December 20, 1999 the squamous neck cancer was removed in a three hour operation at Johns Hopkins. At that point, I researched all information about cancer and determined that the cure rate was 1/2% and that I had a 19% probability of being alive in 5 years. I rejected radiation and took a waiting posture. In May 2000 a biopsy of a mass found at the base of my tongue indicated another squamous cell carcinoma. It was identified by Johns Hopkins as *most probably* the primary tumor. Again, I rejected the recommended 35 radiation treatments as well as radical face and neck surgery.

My research resulted in my desire to use a facility called Hospital Santa Monica, owned by Dr. Kurt Donsbach, Ph.D., if at all possible. I talked to a wonderful lady, Peggy Hanna, and arranged to arrive on May 16, 2000 for cancer therapy. I completed the program on June 7th. Information on Dr. Donsbach and all the treatment protocols may be found on www.donsbach.com and www.hospitalsantamonica.com. Since my return home, I have returned to Johns Hopkins six times for examinations, CT Scans and lab work. Presently there are *no* indications of cancer at all in my body.

My research indicates that cancer is a systemic rather than a localized disease that has cause factors related to environment and nutrition, and therefore, can be cured.

The use of a multi-modal approach to combat a very complex disease was most important. Understanding the relationship between oxygen and the cancer cell is vital. Oxygen therapies are truly a *do no harm* approach. The same cannot be said for radiation nor chemo. It is a gross error on the medical community in the United States to reject studies made in American universities as related to the value of chelation, ozone (O_3), hydrogen peroxide and other proven protocols.

In the United States, cancer is approaching a $180 billion per year industry. As a result of this amount of money, I feel that the pharmaceutical industry controls and guides the direction regarding cancer treatment in America. The American Cancer Society was of no value to me in any respect. The cancer patient must research, direct and assume the position of case manager for his or her self.

ERIKA HUNZIKER
BREAST CANCER

I was diagnosed with breast cancer in November, 2000 and was advised to have surgery immediately. I however, was determined right from the start to follow a natural cure, against the strenuous objections of my doctors. My decision resulted in a course of action utilizing every possible remedy I was able to discover, which included the combination of several therapies. These therapies included various detoxification programs, Far-infrared rays, juicing fasts (including self-grown wheat grass), mega-doses of enzymes and vitamins, high enemas, hot and cold treatments, Immunocal, etc.

The fact that the lump grew much smaller and softer was quite encouraging, but after a full year of self-administered help, a PET scan showed that I was not fully healed. There were still cancer cells present. In February, 2002, I contacted Dr. Ross Hauser of Caring Medical and Rehabilitation Services in Oak Park, Illinois. By June, 2002, after 12 Insulin Potentiation Treatments, with no major side effects, I was declared cancer free! I will continue for the rest of my life to thank and praise my Heavenly Father for his help in making me well again!

It is my faith in God that carried me throughout this ordeal and Dr. Hauser and his staff who became tools in his hands and instruments of his love for my benefit.

ROSELLA RICHMOND
OVARIAN CANCER

It was the summer of 1979; I wasn't feeling like my energetic self. I needed naps in the mid-day. As time went on, I developed a pressure in my right side of the abdominal area, then I got a pain in my right leg that just wouldn't go away. I thought I had a pinched nerve, so I visited a chiropractor. After three treatments he knew I needed to seek other treatments, so he referred me to another doctor. He said to come back Monday, this was on Friday. I couldn't wait until then and now I couldn't walk, sleep or eat. My husband took me to the emergency room on Saturday. After going through the testing to find out the problem, my surgeon informed me at this point they couldn't tell me what was wrong or what parts of my body could be affected. They wanted to know if I would consent to exploratory surgery. I agreed to it. Wednesday, which was the following day, the surgery was performed. After I woke up my husband was there. Tearfully, he told me it was cancer. As we all know — *that never happens to you!*

I took it well because I was positive; I felt better now than when I entered the hospital, and I was still alive after a 3 hour surgery. I knew I was going to get well! That was until my scheduled 25 cobalt treatments were beginning. After 4 of them, I lost five pounds and was so very ill, I felt suicidal. If it hadn't been for my strong belief in God and my wonderful, beautiful family, I wouldn't have hesitated. It was then that I decided to have consultation with my surgeon, who was a super doctor. This appointment was at 2 pm the very same day and time I was supposed to have my 5th cobalt treatment. My surgeon informed me since they had done so much cutting inside me and the 2 lb., very malignant, tumor was wrapped around my kidney area and the tumor broke during surgery, he said I needed all 25 cobalt treatments.

Since I had skipped my 5th cobalt treatment, the nurse

called me to ask why I had skipped my treatment. I said, "They are making me sick." She said, "That's just anxiety. Are you coming tomorrow?" I said, "I don't know." She said, "We don't operate like that, if you don't come tomorrow, we'll give your appointment to someone else." I said, "Thank you." I feel like that was another answer to my prayers, which I had received so many of. The treatment was killing me, not the disease.

The following Thursday I was on my way to Mexico to the "Bio-Medical Clinic" to partake of the "Hoxsey Program." After one visit I became mentally healthy, which is first in the requirement for healing any disease. That clinic gave me *hope*. They put everyone in an individualized program. They tell you what not to eat and drink.

I advise everyone who needs it, to visit the "BioMedical Clinic." I believe it was the most effective part of my healing, along with prayer, positive attitude and loving life! I am in good health after 23 years since being diagnosed with ovarian cancer. I didn't think I'd live for another Christmas, and now I will be celebrating my 24th one.

MARYE BARKER
OVARIAN CANCER

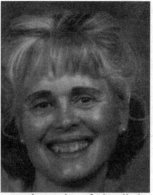

I had complained for a decade of declining health. In May I had a gynecological check and I was told all was fine, but that there were some abnormal cells in pap smear. The doctor refused to do the test again. At the end of June, I could not sit due to rectum pain. I went to a regular doctor, who diagnosed cancer. I had surgery with Dr. Peters in Seattle, and then I started chemotherapy. I had an allergic response to chemo, and was told they would put me on a less effective drug and instead of living 18 months, I would live 14 months. I would end up doing chemo in-hospital on a 24 hour basis. I immediately went to an alternative/immune supportive doctor and have continued that therapy. This doctor, Dr. Douglas Brodie, gave me hope. My general practitioner continues to do Reiki with me and I do massage weekly. I also do daily imaging, and I read everything positive I can. I didn't find cancer support groups very helpful. Support from my friends and family bolsters me everyday.

I believe the most effective part of my healing was immune and family support, plus a good surgeon.

Susan Moss
Breast and Uterine Cancer

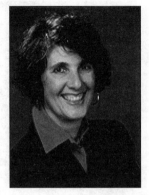

Eleven years ago, I was diagnosed with breast and uterine cancer. It was a cold, gray day in my gynecologist's office, and I remember feeling fear, and a chilly disbelief.

Dr. Furr told me in no uncertain terms, to "see a surgeon." I said, "No." He called me for several days after that. "See a surgeon!" he firmly repeated. Each time, I said, "No."

Finally, he gave in a bit. "Come back in two months!" I said I would and made an appointment with his nurse.

The first thing I did was decide not to cry and not to be a victim, but rather to take action. I joined the YMCA and mapped out a specific work-out program with Mike Cole, a physical therapist. I compiled a 20 point health program (MOTEP) Marathon Olympic Tumor Eradication Prevention Program which covered all areas of my life — spiritual, mental, emotional, diet and exercise. I did this program with all my heart and soul. In 2 months I rid myself of the tumors. It took 7 more months to totally heal and rebuild my body back into health.

I think that believing I could heal myself was the most effective part of my healing. Also, supporting my body in all ways — spiritually, mentally, emotionally, with diet, exercise, group therapy, chanting, prayers and topical natural treatment, plus laughter, juicing, helping others and changing my life.

To further help others, I wrote *Keep Your Breasts!*, which is now in all bookstores in 3 languages to share my program.

RALPH DELL'ANNO
COLON CANCER

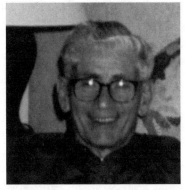

In 1995, I was diagnosed with colon cancer. I was scheduled for colon surgery and went into the hospital with my family, full of confidence I would be fine. They removed one-third of my cancerous colon and I recuperated fine. When I went into to see the doctor after a month, he suggested chemo to keep it under control. I mentioned to the doctor that I decided not to have chemo and was going to go to an alternative route. He told me he wouldn't be responsible for the results, and I said, "Fine, I'll take responsibility for this choice." I went to International Bio Care Hospital, stayed a week and came home to continue vitamins and whatever else the program called for. In 1998, after another colonoscopy, they found 2 more polyps of cancer. They removed them and I went down to Mexico again for two days. I have continued with my program ever since, and have been cancer free for over 4 1/2 years now.

I believe the most effective part of my healing was first off, my faith in God. Also, trust and faith in the loving doctors at the International Bio Care Hospital in Mexico — The care and loving ways and assurance — "You can do it!" Also, the support and love from my family, who were with me all the way. I accepted the will of God and I won!

Another effective part of my healing was my friend and mentor Louise Rotala who lived in Loveland, Colorado. She told me that a few of our friends had colon cancer, had done the operation and then resumed their healing with alternative medicine by going to Bio Care Hospital. I did not hesitate a moment and I have been free of cancer since 1998.

Believe in yourself and don't allow doctors to take away your choice of making your own decisions, of being cancer free!

MARY HARRINGTON
MELANOMA

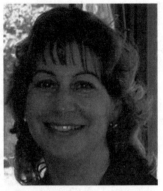

I was scheduled for surgery in January, 1996, for a bartholin's and perineal neoplasia. However, they found a 5-6 centimeter malignant melanoma tumor. Because of the amount of tissue and a small amount of rectum removed, a colostomy was performed. I went into a minor surgery and woke up with my life changed forever. I was on morphine, and emotionally I was in shock and very scared. Both doctors gave me a poor prognosis at that time; they told me to just go live my life. I was determined to do whatever it took to live. I was 39 years old and had two children in high school.

I went through 25 treatments of radiation and 30 days of interferon fed intravenously; thereafter, I gave myself injections three times a week for 3 months until a CT scan showed the melanoma had metastasis. I had two 2-3 centimeter tumors on the left side with another small one on my right side of my liver. This was 8 months after my first diagnosis. I had two liver biopsies. The first was negative; I thought God had healed me through prayers. My oncologist wanted another biopsy. The second was positive. I was exhausted and weak; my weight had dropped from 125 to 114 pounds. I couldn't eat or even take vitamins due to the pain in my stomach. I was pale and very depressed. The interferon causes this. I also worked in a full-time job through all of this. I prayed more, cried more, but I continued to trust in God no matter what happened. It was what I repeated to my children constantly. "Trust in God no matter what happens."

I was then given 3 to 6 months to live. My oncologist offered chemo treatments to possibly give me a few more months if my body responded. He said with enthusiasm that I could maybe live up to 9 months. I had to do the hardest thing I've ever done; I had to go home and tell my children. My daughter cried, "It's not fair, you're supposed to be there when I get married and when I have my first baby." My son went silent.

I had two children and I wanted to finish raising them. I was desperate to live. I had a friend who looked on the Internet and found the Gerson Institute. He looked into everything, spoke with some former patients, the doctors, staff and would not give up. He would call me daily. I was just so hesitant — medical treatment in Tijuana, Mexico? I thank God for him. I spoke with about 6 patients, one who was in the same condition as I was, stage 4 melanoma, and they were all still alive years later.

I had worked in the medical field for 11 years in the office; alternative treatments were really new to me. I was very skeptical and uncertain, but the patients are the ones who convinced me. One of the patients told me, there are a lot of us out there (free of cancer). I figured, if they could do it, I could.

The experience I had there was a great one. My husband stayed with me during the duration of the stay and we met people from all over the world, all wanting to be healed of cancer. My doctor was patient, understanding and just so confident about the diet. The diet was not easy, but I was a very determined person. I am also a Christian and did a lot of praying and soul searching. I went to cancer support groups. I had regular massages and chiropractic care. I also did aromatherapy. I read a lot of books on positive things. I surrounded myself with positive people in a positive environment. I did what I could to relieve myself of stress. I did whatever I thought would help heal my body. I had to clean a lot of vegetables for the diet so we had what we called *carrot cleaning parties*, where family and friends would come over for a few hours and help clean vegetables every weekend.

Ten months on the diet I had my first scan that showed clear. I continued the diet and did it for a full 2 years. I still see my oncologist regularly and have CT scans yearly and I am still in remission. My diet is normal other than I do not eat meat other than fish. I still use my juicer and buy organic produce. I take vitamins and a few supplements. I work out, lifting weights to build up my bones, since I had bone loss from the radiation.

Based on what I know now, I would have skipped the cancer treatments I did here in the states and went straight to the Gerson Institute. I still have side effects that I have to deal with due to the radiation I had. The treatments I did made me weaker rather than better. After coming home from Mexico, I went to see my oncologist and told him what I was doing, and that I still needed him to see me and order lab work for this diet. He recommended that I do not do the diet, as he felt it was harmful and he noted it in my chart. I chose to do it anyway. I am now known as his *amazing patient*. I am alive with a future. I have since seen both my children graduate, my daughter get married, and I have become a grandmother. I have been in eleven different states and travel as much as possible, and I try not to take life for granted.

BARBARA CHARIS
VAGINAL TUMOR

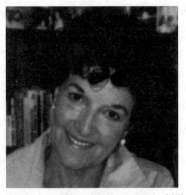

My fourth child was born May 8th, 1976. When I went in for the standard six week check-up, I asked the doctor to check thoroughly, because I was in agony. Just walking brought tears to my eyes. I was in so much pain. He did a thorough examination and told me that I had a fast growing tumor, which needed to be surgically removed.

I trusted my O.B., but I went to another doctor for a second opinion. The second doctor said that he would give me no guarantees if I didn't have the tumor removed immediately. I refused to set up a date for surgery. I told him that I was going to go home and pray. He said I shouldn't pray too long.

Two and a half months later, I paid him for a second visit to show him that my tumor was gone. I wanted to tell him what I did, but he wasn't interested. All he said was it occurred from *spontaneous remission*.

When I found out that I had the tumor, I asked both medical doctors if they knew anything about *autolysis*. I had read in my nutritional research (which I had been into for 15 years at this point) about the ability of the human body to get rid of any excess material, such as a tumor by not giving it the *fuel* it needed to grow. Both doctors told me that they knew nothing about autolysis.

After my second visit to the doctor, I did go home and pray. I asked for guidance, and in less than a week a book came into my hands, which gave me some answers. It was entitled *The Vegetarian Guide to Diet and Salad* by Norman W. Walker, Ph.D. Dr. Walker was an esteemed health consultant who had written about ten books and was a living example. He lived well over 100 years of age, working and writing until he died. There are documents I have seen which show his date of birth as 1876 and he died in 1985. He knew a great deal about health.

I followed his dietary suggestions, which were to go completely raw foods (fruits and vegetables only). He also said to eliminate all stress and to get sufficient rest. He said to get natural sunlight on a daily basis. Above all, I was to keep my mind attuned to the Creator, and trust in the Creator's ability to heal me.

It is now 26 years later and the above tumor never returned. It was completely eliminated with my raw fruit and vegetables dietary program and the other changes. I used no medication or treatments.

In 1988, another smaller tumor manifested on my chest. It took me just weeks to get rid of that growth, too. I looked in the food diary that I kept and when I calculated how much raw honey I was using, I couldn't believe it. I was using about 5 lbs. every 3 weeks in my herb teas. When I realized this, I stopped the honey completely, and stayed with only raw foods for about ten weeks. And then the growth I had was gone.

I went at first to a doctor to ask for advice and was told that it should be surgically removed or I was asking for trouble. It was a nasty multi-colored raspberry-like growth, and was the size of about two large grapes. Three months later there was only a very smooth pink surface and nothing to indicate that a growth had ever been there.

I didn't waste my time paying for another doctor's visit. I didn't want to hear about *spontaneous remission* again.

I came to the conclusion that cancerous growths are created by eating excess protein, fat and carbohydrates. These in abundance are fuels, which trigger off growths in the human body.

After I got rid of the first tumor, I wrote to the M.D. Anderson Tumor Hospital in Texas. I told the hancho exactly what I did in order to eliminate my tumor. He got my information ... that is for sure. However, the information was not used the way I told him in my letter. The people there used dairy protein to make the tumor grow further, so there would be more tumor to *kill* with their chemo. I was not a subscriber to "Let's Live" magazine, but somehow the Creator guided me to pick up a copy randomly and peruse it. In it was an article about the Anderson hospital using the dairy protein. I bought it and have shared the info with thousands of people over the last 20+ years.

I need to add that after the second tumor, I stopped sunbathing for about 13 years, as I started to become concerned with the amount of skin damage which was occurring on my body. Since 1988, I had spent 54 years sunbathing. The skin on my chest was looking rather leathery and my face was wrinkling.

Two months ago I started doing a limited amount of daily sunbathing, because the best source of Vitamin D is made directly by sunbathing. I do have very strong bones and I want to avoid osteoporosis. Without Vitamin D, and the best is natural sunlight, the body will deteriorate. Calcium and other minerals work synergistically with Vitamin D.

I believe the most effective part of my healing was asking the Creator for guidance. The Creator has the answers we need. Right after I asked, the answers came in the form of Dr. Norman Walker's book. I totally trust in the Master Physician with all my heart, mind and soul. I have seen other incredible healings, because of my trust.

Natural, simple truth is the best. There is no man-made product or treatment which can bring about a cure. We have to discover the cause and eliminate the cause. If we lived right, thought right, ate right and were attuned to our Maker, we would never become ill.

Every problem that I ever encountered was overcome simply by eliminating the cause — from arthritis to cancer to migraines, soar throats, etc. One does not build natural immunity by using vaccines. I was healthy, because I was not going for any vaccinations or using medicine, not even aspirin. My body had the ability to heal, because I was trying to eat right, even before these things happened. As Hosea 4: 6 stated, "My people perish through lack of knowledge."

KAY KOCISKO
OVARIAN CANCER

I'd like to start this account with the return of my cancer, which was April 2001. Prior to that, I got my original diagnosis March 24, 2000, but that seemed like a *closed case* because surgical removal of the left ovary and tube. They thought they got it all. No clinical therapy was required, and life seemed nearly unchanged for me for a whole year. A physical in Oct. 2000 said everything was normal, so I kept my routines intact and prayerfully (although a bit apprehensively) went on with life.

Then, in March, 2001, I had serious bloating of my abdominal area and a nagging kidney pain — all too reminiscent of my symptoms a year earlier.

A CT scan and blood work revealed that my ovarian cancer had returned and had metastasized in a way that was inoperable. The oncologist at Cleveland Clinic determined the only possible treatment would be chemo.

Knowing a number of people that suffered immense side-effects (and some died) during chemo, my husband and I decided chemo was NOT an option. We then researched alternative methods and narrowed down our options by what we could afford. Next we (and many others) prayed for us to make the right choice.

We decided to go with a detox, strict diet and supplement plan with the help of a nutritional counselor. After 3 months, my tumor area had shrunk back almost to normal size. My energy was low, but my general health was good and I was suffering no pain. By mid-summer, I started to experience edema in my legs, and another very strange thing happened.

My fingertips began to have circulation problems. They became purple, cold and began to turn black. I later learned this was capillary clotting due to the tremendous amount of protein in my blood, from the cancer. The fingertip tissue was becoming necrotic (dying). We knew we had to do something immediately. We got help from a circulation specialist in Canada and weathered that frightening problem, which took 6 months to reverse and grow new fingertip tissue.

During the winter (January 2002), the swelling in my tumor area started to increase. Even though I had experienced a burst of energy during the holidays, I was completely exhausted by mid-January, 2002. Edema in my legs was worse and I was now experiencing a fluid build-up (ascites) in my lower and mid-stomach areas. My breathing became more difficult.

At this time, my nutritional counselor had found out about the Young for Life Medical Clinic in Athens, Ohio, which was only a three hour drive from our home. My counselor recommended I check it out ASAP. After talking with the doctor there and more prayerful consideration we decided to try it for 3 weeks.

The first thing done was to get a CT Scan and a number of lab tests to see "where I was." The doctor said I had the largest tumor mass of anyone he'd ever seen! The tumor mass extended from the pelvic area to the base of my heart. Immediately they started me on IPT treatment, which is a unique way of administering low-dose chemotherapy. A description of this method of low-dose chemotherapy, which has virtually no side-effects can be found on the clinic's website: {youngforlife.com}.

At the end of 3 weeks, a comparative CT Scan was done and the tumor had shrunk by 40%! Wow! My leg and abdomen swelling had decreased considerably and I was feeling my energy coming back. Praise God! Since the results were so incredibly good, it was obvious we should continue treatment here.

The next CT scan (5-02) showed overall tumor reduction of 80%. We knew I was definitely improving! My energy was increasing steadily and I began to regain my normal weight. My June CT scan showed further tumor reduction and only a few enlarged lymph nodes left.

We know this is all God's doing, and we are forever

grateful for His awesome mercy! We are also incredibly grateful to all the people who have been there during all this to pray and share their love with me and my family. I am currently anticipating my next CT scan and look forward to the completion of my treatment.

My experiences at the Young for Life Medical Clinic have been *so* positive! The doctor and his staff are very caring and provide individual attention for each of the patient's needs. Also, the patients feel drawn to encourage and support one another. Our common goal of healing and seeing one another's progress generates a joyful energy at the Young for Life Clinic!

I believe I was healed by God's compassionate love for me demonstrated through my husband and so many people, and IPT treatment at Young for Life Medical Clinic in Athens, Ohio.

JUDY DAVIS
COLON CANCER

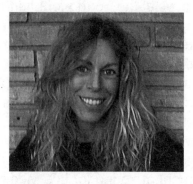

It was a beautiful day in April, 1992, but I had a bad tummy ache. Nearing the end of my Isla Mujeres trip, on my plane trip out of Cancun, I felt very uncomfortable and bloated. I got home in Santa Barbara on Monday and called my doctor. He suggested an enema. No success. By Wednesday he scheduled a colonic and after two hours, still nothing had moved. Now I had a fever, which was rare for me, so Thursday he scheduled an upper GI series at a hospital lab. (I'd actually wanted an MRI, but what did I know?) All day they tried to get photos and after 3 - 8 oz. glasses of barium my stomach was quite distended and I was in agonizing pain. 'You're a keeper," they said and I was admitted to the hospital late Thursday afternoon and given Demerol for the pain. Friday morning I vaguely remember being wheeled down to the lab for a lower GI which merely showed I was blocked and needed immediate exploratory surgery that afternoon. Though still very drugged from the continued Demerol, I wanted to talk to my admitting family doctor for an explanation, but on a Friday afternoon they couldn't find him. The surgeon and anesthesiologist were quite irate with me saying it was imperative I have immediate exploratory surgery, that the 'operating theatre' was available that afternoon. My retort, "... is this for your convenience or my life?" I remember the anesthesiologist indignantly stomping out of the room. Without the benefit of friends or family or even my own doctor and still in a drugged haze, I finally succumbed and signed the release forms.

I awoke Saturday noon with a large incision down my belly and my warned parents there by my bedside. The results? Well, I'd had a large tumor they removed, along with about 2/4 of my large intestine during a resection. I'd better speak to the cancer specialist. My reply? "A tumor? Did you get it all?" Answer, "Yes, but you need to speak to the cancer specialist." So I knew something was up. I was to stay in the hospital for a week ... no cancer specialist there... waiting for a week, wondering....

The next day, Sunday afternoon, still in the hospital and only two days after surgery, they took me off IV and brought my first whole meal. When I lifted the lid and saw a roast beef dinner I was appalled! Common sense told me my first meal of whole food after a major resection should be easy, like soup broth but the nurses just looked at the chart and said, "No, your doctor said you can eat this." I had them bring me soup. No one would tell me anything but the visiting faces of family and friends for the week I stayed hospitalized were friendly, encouraging, but worried. Did they know something I didn't?

About 10 days after the surgery, the cancer specialist said I had colon cancer. I took a tape recorder, which I later read he'd put in his notes as a caution to other medical professionals. Geez!!! I just wanted to document some probably very foreign technical data from a specialist I'd only get to talk to a short while and they were already branding me 'difficult'. He said the biopsy showed 52 nodes and 7 of them tested positive — rated Duke C-3. Those sounded like good odds to me but he said, "No, you have maybe a 17% chance of survival and you need to start chemotherapy right away." He explained the process. My first immediate, internal response was of a burning going into my veins, and I told him I'd think about it.

Friends put me in touch with John Fink and his book *Third Opinion*, a manual of clinics and therapies around the world that he and his wife put together after losing their daughter to cancer. At the time, Tijuana was the cancer capitol of the world, so I selected about 10 clinics to visit. Without much money and clearly needing to do something right away I expedited by search by first calling my psychically gifted sister-in-law, Mary, who gave me a crystal healing ceremony prior to medical treatment. But first, over the phone, I asked her to give me an objective, psychic reading on just the numbers 1-10 (I'd selected 10 clinics to visit) to help guide and expedite my upcoming one day tour in Tijuana. Without her reading I would have given up on number 5 clinic, as it had moved and I couldn't find it. But with such a strong *hit* from Mary on number 5, my driver kept looking for it, and we found it very late in the day. It was the one. They accepted me on a promise of funding and I went back home to pack my bags for a six week, outpatient stay.

Dr. Gustavo Andrade was my principal doctor and the main therapy was from Dr. Lawrence Burton's Immuno-Augmentative Therapy (based in the Bahamas) along with shark cartilage enemas and mega-doses of vitamins.

Well, it was quite an experience. Funding came from generous contributions of family and friends. My mom even sold her wedding ring for me! So I set off on an adventure. First I stayed at some border motel then later got myself a cheap, little apartment in La Playa (the beach section of Tijuana) and a $10 bike and would pedal over to the clinic every morning about 7:30 for blood work. Drawing my blood each morning enabled them to analyze what combination of blood serum I should have and monitor me through the six weeks. About 10 a.m they'd start giving me from 7-12 subcutaneous injections I'd give myself every hour throughout the day. Hating shots and needles, this was by far the most difficult part of my therapy, but I did it. Dr. Andrade was very warm and friendly and always had plenty of time to explain everything I wanted to know. "There's no silver bullet, Judy, so we're going to do several things along with the self injections and you're going to be fine!" His staff was wonderful and I met many, dear friends that were fellow patients there. Upon departure, I was given customized injections to take daily for three months until my return.

In late September, I went back for more blood analysis and monitoring, got my needles and headed home for another three months. January was my last trip and it went well for me but due to NAFTA some clinics, including mine, were shut down. Fortunately, Dr. Andrade continued to help any and all patients he could.

Looking back, I was very fortunate. After my surgery I never suffered any pain like so many others I saw in Tijuana. At first, hating the hourly injections, my skin reacted to that fear by puffing up right after my shot, bleeding, bruising and hurting. Within a month I could inject myself while walking down the street without breaking stride! And no bruise, no blood and no pain. Why? My body was so used to it and I had no fear, no trepidations. However, after a year of daily (every hour) injections my body began to speak to me; with bruising, bleeding and pain. It just seemed to say it was really sick and tired of being a pin-cushion. So I stopped all therapy but continued, at home, my regular checkups and annual sigmoidoscopies. I paid better attention to my diet but most of all my thoughts and feelings. The doctors all had concluded that my tumor had taken at least 2 years to grow, so I was able to realize that what I had started in my personal life about 2 years ago had a lot to do with it.

In my adult life I've always believed one creates their own reality, so if I *caused* my tumor I could *un-cause* it. I had never believed, or even considered, my "17% prognosis". I was concerned enough to seek some kind of therapy which educated me in cancer treatments outside of the A.M.A.'s strict guidelines and narrow options. Had I done nothing, who knows? I might still have succeeded. Apart from the great adventure and the many friends along the way, I concluded that intent and attitude are the single most important tools one can ever have in conquering any of life's trials.

And now it's ten years later, almost to the day. I just returned from Tijuana and a re-examination from my dear Dr. Andrade. What a pleasure to see him again! All of this time, these past ten years, I'd only seen American doctors for my cancer check-ups. Even though I've been diligent regarding my health, none of these American doctors have the decades of experience with alternative and integrative medicine that these foreign doctors have. What a huge relief to be under his care again and to get a clean bill of health! And all of my tests and complete examination were a fraction of the cost I'd pay in the U.S.!

After my exam Dr. Andrade personally drove me on a tour to meet his top-notch associate doctors and visit the clinics. I had a chance to speak privately with some of his current patients and it just re-affirmed my opinion of him. One British man had nothing but praise and told me Dr. Andrade had once driven from Mexico City to San Diego (many hundreds of miles) just to pick up a critical patient at the airport. Just a few months ago I also learned that my dear doctor had designed the protocol and treatment that saved the life of Max Factor's son Donald. We ended the day with a scrumptious dinner prepared by his lovely wife, Luc Maria, a published and working nutritionist.

Yes, I know now more than ever I'm in good hands. From a string of events on the day my U.S. doctor gave me only a small chance of survival to psychic readings and sheer determination, I am living proof that anyone can survive cancer. Because of this amazing 'chapter' in my life I've been asked to write this chapter in Bliss' book. She met me through the magazine I work with called "Natural Beauty and Health." They published my cancer story in their Fall 2002 issue and I just designed a new section called "Alternative Healing" in the 2003 spring issue that's dedicated to miraculous healing stories from patients, clinics and doctors worldwide. It's been a whirlwind for me to meet so many wonderful new friends again in the healing circles. Even more incredible has been revisiting Dr. Andrade and his associated to see what's currently happening in Mexico.

Today I'm armed with knowledge, experience and the best doctors and clinics available on the planet. Now it's my great opportunity to give back. There is hope. One always has many choices and due to both dedicated doctors and patients alike there is a way.

I hope my story and all the stories in this book find their way into the minds, hearts and bodies of those in need. I welcome anyone to contact me if they wish information and support. Yes! Life is an adventure and it's great to be living it.

JOHN LALLO
BRAIN TUMOR

My story starts with a number of things that happened to me when I came home from a vacation from Hawaii. I started being forgetful. I'd leave on the gas on the stove. I'd leave water running in the sink. I'd leave the front door open all night. Then I'd forget appointments. I was really tired also. Then my legs got rubbery and I fell. Then I had bath room accidents. My wife took me to the urgent care after a few weeks and I fell there so they put me in the hospital for a CAT scan. The doc said I had a brain tumor and it was cancer. Within 2 weeks I was operated on and they took a fifty cent round tumor out of my head. Told me it was grade 3 autosycoma. But after the lab work it came back grade 4. The doc said I'd have 1 year if I did chemo and radiation. My wife looked for other treatments. My friends came to my house and helped us as soon as I came home. They brought Essiac tea with them and I started that right away and have been on that ever since.

My wife talked to my son who works for UPS, and his friend told him that oxygen helped her father who had lung cancer, so he got the phone number of person that helped him and my wife called and talked to him. Also my wife got a book from the library and this backed up what was told to us by Keith, the man we buy the Hydroxygen Plus from. So I started this, as well as MSM, and changed my diet to no sugar or meat or white flour. I decided not to fry my brains and the doctor is shocked I'm still alive. I have had 2 MRI's and there has been no cancer so far growing back. The MRI doc called me and asked what we are doing because he was concerned and told my wife I should be dead. He also wants to see me in 3 months. So September is my 9th month check up. We are now selling the Hydroxygen Plus, and we try to help any one that calls us.

I believe having a positive outlook is very important

also the most important is a belief in God and prayer. I also had good support from my family and friends and spiritual brothers. It is important to stick to a good program. Not hit and miss. You must do your research. The answers are out there, but you must have faith.

TERRY FRANCO
BREAST CANCER

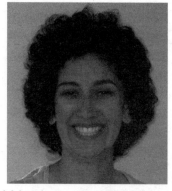

When I was told I had cancer, all I felt was great sense of peace go through my body that everything was going to be fine. Many people fear this disease, but I knew this was a gift from God, and that I was to experience a special journey and to live to tell others about this.

My search began with options of choosing traditional or alternative treatments. Since a biopsy was performed and the tumor was disturbed, the doctors were now pressing me to have a lumpectomy with radiation as soon as possible. I knew time was my side! I knew in my heart that surgery was not the way for me.

I began with a deep cleansing of my body's toxins. I did a 30-day cleanse, changed my nutrition, and exercised. I visited the Young Life Research Clinic in Utah for one week and began a regime of essential oils, colonics, biofeedback, and started a liquid fast which I continued for 15 days. I had amazing energy levels and loved it. I also worked with Dr. Leeder in clearing my emotions and using applied kinesiology for my nutrition and many other things. This is key for any recovery.

I then returned to the conventional doctors after three months. They listed my options as doing a mastectomy with chemotherapy and suggesting removal of my ovaries as well. I felt like a fish being skinned out. I told the doctors that I was going to continue my alternative option. Needless to say, they were not pleased. Remember this is your body and you have to take responsibility for it, and learn to heal it. We all need our immune system to live and be healthy. Chemotherapy is a poison that I couldn't choose to put in my body or anyone else's.

I started to search the Internet and found many alternative options. I kept hearing about the American Metabolic Institute in Mexico and Dr. Rubio. I spoke with patients who had great successes, so I went there for a consultation. I learned his protocol of taking a piece of the tumor to make a vaccine that is reinserted back into the body to reverse the cancer cells. It is called an auto-immune vaccine. Within a week, I was back at the clinic beginning my daily treatment, which included IV's, ozone, rife, coffee and shark enemas, vitamins and minerals, color therapy, juicing and good healthy organic food. The hospital was very warm and welcoming by staff and patients. I had a very positive experience and highly recommend it to anyone. I returned home 13 days later to my wonderful family and continue to do my home program and am doing very well. My cancer has remained removed from my body and will stay that way. I continue my healthy lifestyle and show people they can do it too.

I feel that bringing together mind, body and spirit is key to healing your body and keeping your immune system at its best. We all have options and each one of us is given a choice and has free will.

I believe my personal belief in power of prayer and bringing in God's light throughout my body, my daily devotions and meditating was the key to my recovery. It was so soothing to listen to positive tapes and music. I was given a great book titled *The Bible Cure for Cancer,* by Don Colbert M.D., which gave me the faith, trust and strength to keep my mind in line with God and to never take my eyes off him. Miracles can happen, and I know God let me remain here to continue to tell others what is possible!

DAVID EMERSON
MULTIPLE MYELOMA

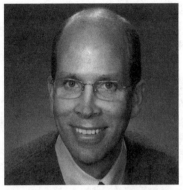

I was born 12/24/59. There was no family history of cancer. At the age of 34, I was very healthy. The only factor that I can think of was extreme stress of job.

I was diagnosed with single plasmacytoma in C5 of my neck. Local radiation was the only therapy done at that time. It was full-blown multiple myeloma about a year later. I had 5 courses of VAD (a combination treatment of vincristine, doxorubicin and dexamethasone), 2 courses of cytoxin and peripheral blood stem cell transplant, all in 1995. I had a bone marrow transplant (BMT) at the Ireland Cancer Center at University Hospitals of Cleveland.

I married Dawn White on 9/14/96. Dawn was my best friend, lover and primary care giver through all the above. I could not have gone through any of this without her. I had first occurrence 6 weeks after our marriage. The oncologist recommended local radiation. A radiologist named Don Shina recommended that I collect and freeze some sperm. This proved to be a wonderful recommendation.

Local radiation temporarily staved off the multiple myeloma, but the next 10 months showed signs of growing problem. Over the course of the next 11 months, my HMO assigned me 4 different oncologists. Over the next four years, my HMO would fight my therapy every step of the way.

In September of 1997, my oncologist recommended palliative care, having exhausted all other options, in her opinion. This was a nice way of prescribing pain management drugs until I died.

I began a cancer therapy called *antineoplaston therapy* in November of 1997. I underwent 10 months of the liquid form of the therapy, and then 7 months of the capsule form. My disease stabilized and eventually went away. After eight years since my diagnosis, I am in complete remission.

I believe the most important part of my healing was the realization that I needed to take complete control of my healing process. After three years of following my conventional oncologists recommendations and having nothing to show for it, other than a host of debilitating side effects, I was forced to take control of my therapy and pursued many forms of healing. The list of health improving pursuits included giving up alcohol and caffeine, about 50% raw foods diet, homeopathy, a variety of herbs and supplements, and an excellent exercise regimen to name a few. The *debulking* of the antineoplaston therapy was critical to it all.

Multiple myeloma is an obscure and unique form of cancer that requires each patient to learn as much as he/she can about his/her own disease and the available forms of therapy. My journey was long and arduous and doesn't translate well here. The current state of modern HMO medicine and the uniqueness and severity of multiple myeloma requires that each patient take control of his/her own therapy.

I would be more than happy to talk to anyone interested in anything about the above information.

MARK OLSZTYN
BRAIN TUMOR

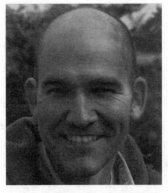

My story begins in late March of 1991 in Davis, California. At around 3 o'clock in the morning I was awakened by paramedics. My fiancee had called them and reported that I was having a seizure in my sleep. When I saw the two rain-drenched paramedics and the concern on Belinda's face, I thought, "This can only be a nightmare."

I was transported to a nearby hospital where a CAT scan was done, revealing either a contusion or a tumor. The doctor wasn't sure which. An MRI confirmed it was a tumor located in the left frontal lobe. It seemed to be well circumscribed and easily operable, so surgery seemed to be the natural course to follow.

It was removed on April 4, 1991 and diagnosed as a low-grade malignant tumor: an oligodendroastrocytoma grade 1. Post-operative treatment was ruled unnecessary, and I was told I needed only to have an MRI every six months. I was told that there was a 50% probability of it coming back—the toss of a coin. I was also told that if it did come back, it would be much more malignant, although I don't remember having been told that particular fact.

I became obsessed with my odds, literally making bets against a recurrence dozens of times a day to alleviate the stress between scans, which were the ultimate arbiter in my life. Though I never actually tossed a coin, these *bets* were always slightly hedged in my favor, such as, "If I can walk the entire length of this fallen log without losing my balance it means that I'm going to be okay." I nonetheless lost a few such wagers in my desperate search for some sign that everything was going to be all right.

The time approaching my next scan was when I really began to break down. I had found work in the news graphics department at a television station in Sacramento a few months after my recovery. My job was preparing the backgrounds, maps, and over-the-shoulder imagery for the six and nine o'clock news. It could be either exhilarating or hellishly stressful. It all depended on the presence or absence of glitches. Quite naturally to me, these glitches became a part of my betting scheme. Because I hadn't shared my recent medical history when I applied for the position six months earlier, no one at work quite understood why I took my job so seriously.

The lag time between the scan and receiving the results by phone at work was what I found almost unbearable. It could come at any moment from two to five days after the scan. Good news or bad. The phone would ring and I would jump. It was this stress, which on two occasions actually brought on migraine headaches, necessitating my having to go home, that eventually drove me to stop getting scanned altogether, and thus began my long and nearly successful process of denial.

I left California and headed to Connecticut to begin a new life in the Masters program in Graphic Design at Yale. I even contemplated changing my name. I wanted every aspect of my cancer to be behind me once and for all. I would not talk about it. I would not allow others to know about it. Only my fiance knew and understood my reasons for the denial, however flawed they were.

In May of 1995, I graduated Magna Cum Laude and, with our healthy new baby girl in tow and our nuptials decreed, I accepted a position in Watertown, Massachusetts working for a studio specializing in international television branding. It was rewarding, but required long hours and frequent travel. It seemed I was away from home most of the time, but it was exactly where I thought I always wanted to be — married with children, doing creative work in a nice suit, and traveling to places like New York, Los Angeles and Chicago to pitch ideas to entertainment industry executives. By January of 1997, we had a new healthy baby boy and bought a new car. All my dreams seemed right within my grasp until Monday, March 17th — Saint Patrick's Day.

At the persistent urging of a close friend at work (the only person other than my wife who knew about my six years of denial), I consented to getting another scan. The results came back positive the following Monday. A tumor was found in the same location (left frontal lobe) but it was bigger this time: five centimeters instead of the previous three.

On April 7th, I was operated on again. This time it was to remove what was thought to be a Glioblastoma multiforme, or GBM. I met with the chief surgeon and a cadre of specialists two weeks after the operation to hear the diagnosis and, since I had to ask, prognosis. "It all depends on how you take the treatment, Mark," said the surgeon. The treatment he was recommending was standard: 33 rounds of radiation followed by one year of chemotherapy and then, "Hope for the best." Somehow I instinctively knew that hope alone would not be enough this time. I had a fight in front of me and I was going to use any and every means available to win.

At first I was undiscerning, reasoning that fate or God or whatever had placed me in this predicament would also guide me out. I needed merely to do whatever came to me. The very first resource was a package sent to me by my father containing three bottles of Poly-MVA accompanied by a sheaf of information about the product. I browsed the literature and found it convincing in its claim to be a nontoxic cancer-fighting nostrum specific to brain tumors. Poly-MVA's alleged ability to bypass the blood-brain barrier and attack only those cells that are operating anaerobically seemed questionable at first, but the scientific aspect of the writing, which included many charts and diagrams and a patent application, was persuasive enough to get me to try it. There were no sales pitches and, at that time, very little anecdotal testimony to the efficacy of the product, so I proceeded on blind faith and my father's encouragement.

To this regimen I added many others. Some, like Essiac tea and a truly awful tasting Chinese herbal remedy, I tried only once. Shark cartilage, frozen bovine thymus concentrate, mega doses of vitamin C, frankincense essential oil applied to the feet, and super-oxygenated water were also, at one time or another, a part of my approach before, during and after radiation and chemotherapy. These alternative means of fighting cancer all had one thing in common. They gave me a sense of control over my disease. By going outside of what I perceived as the acknowledged shortcomings of conventional medicine's *slash, burn and poison* approach, I felt I was restoring my health even as the radiation and cytotoxins were trying to tear it down.

I decided that it was in my best interest to discontinue my chemotherapy after four out of six rounds. After the second round of PCV (Procarbazine, CCNU—a compound of several different drugs, and Vincristine) I had contracted pertussis, more commonly known as whooping cough and, in the process, lost 25 pounds. I had never felt so sick in my life and began to question, for the first time, the role of conventional (i.e.: allopathic) medicine in my recovery. I had accepted that the surgery was necessary and felt that the radiation follow-up was well-advised, but neither of them had made me physically ill like I was now. I was violently coughing and vomiting while spiking a high fever. After I lost all sensation in my toes, it became clear that I was being eaten alive by chemicals and if I didn't stop soon, I might never fully recover from the damage to my bones and internal organs.

I stayed with the therapy for two more rounds, reasoning that by crossing the half-way point, I will have received enough PCV to do the job. At some point during the fourth round, I received Ralph Moss's *Questioning Chemotherapy* from a friend. Dr. Moss's book informed me that, in the case of brain tumors at least, chemotherapy is a mere palliative; something to add a few months or years to patient's life, but not the cure it can be with some other types of cancers. I found his work and writing to be unbiased, dispassionate and scientifically based; my decision to stop chemotherapy was therefore an informed one. Some months after I had quit, I spoke to the nurse who had administered the intravenous portion of my chemotherapy about my decision and was shocked to hear her say that, in her opinion, radiation is many times more effective in treating brain cancer than chemo. "With something like a GBM," she said, "doctors generally just throw everything at it."

This pell-mell approach seemed to typify conventional medicine's methodology with regard to cancer. After surgery as an option has been exhausted, bombard the patient with radiation and cytotoxins to the point of near physical collapse and hope that the cancer sustained more damage than the patient. Alternative medicine, as I understand it, sees cancer as an opportunistic invader that preys upon weakened immune systems. By strengthening the body's own defenses, say many alternative doctors, diseases like cancer can be controlled and even eliminated entirely.

In addition to the vitamins and tonics I was ingesting, I also practiced the following: yoga; forgiveness; guided meditation and visualization (Christine Northrup during my chemo phase; Joan Borysenko's *Meditations for Self Healing and Inner Power* for gratitude to my body; and, most significantly, Louise Hay's wonderfully soothing *Subliminal Healing* for overall wellness); Qigong; Christian prayer and plain old gratitude. I went to healing services, Reiki therapists, psychotherapists and support groups. I attended wellness seminars and applied to my life just about all I could absorb from M.D. gurus like Bernie Siegel, Andrew Weil and Deepak Chopra. Siegel's book, *Love, Medicine and Miracles* was especially helpful in the very beginning to inspire hope. I would recommend reading that book and Louise Hay's tape to anyone facing this crisis.

I feel that each and every choice I made over the last six years has contributed to my recovery, and I have retained all that I need to retain from them and no longer need to adhere so strictly to their protocols. The only holdover is a tablespoon of freshly ground flax seed in my cereal (for the Omega-3 fatty acids) and teaspoon of Poly-MVA straight with a water chaser every morning. I continue to get a scan every four months and my anxiety levels are gradually diminishing. Fatigue remains a constant companion, however, but I have come to accept that as part of my life.

Although I find nothing particularly heroic about my fight against cancer, I will concede that my journey to recovery shares one aspect of the mythological hero. In their battles against great odds, superior numbers, or superior size they must lose something of value, be it an eye or a kingdom. Two operations and 33 rounds of radiation have left their scars; I have lost my ability to solve complex problems in a systematic way, which was exactly what I used to do for a living. You won't find me feeling sorry for myself, though, because the rewards of being a full-time father and helping the many cancer patients who have contacted me is more fulfilling than anything I have yet imagined.

I believe the most effective part of my healing was the change in attitude from victim to victor which had its origins in Bernie Siegel's book and was bolstered by Louise Haye's tape. To this I must add that hearing about *miracle* recoveries on a semi-regular basis from the Poly-MVA community certainly encourages the hope that I will survive this, too.

Catherine "Kay" Bevan
Ovarian/Endometrial

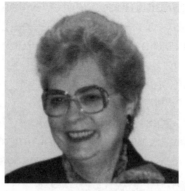

Actually, death was not on my mind in 1989 when I ended my satisfying but exhausting 30-year career as a primary-grade teacher. What with public budget constraints and societal changes, teaching had become increasingly stressful and retirement promised a rewarding change. My new life was to include extensive travel and a carefree existence in a new home located just 50 miles southeast of our former hometown of Tucson. The mountainous region of Sonoita, Arizona can only be described as seductive. Largely a smooth, golden grassland, it is punctuated with enough vigorous features to provide delightful vistas at every turn. But this idyllic setting was blurred by the Grim Reaper's shadow.

The abdominal pressure was fleeting, as was the subsequent pain. But as the Fall of '91 progressed, so did the symptoms, which were strange and unexpected. My internist at the time seemed mystified and thought medications I had been taking for menopausal problems were suddenly backfiring. He seemed to avoid going any further until May of 1992, when the pain became disabling. Finally, referral to a highly respected gynecologist and a resultant sonogram picked up the pace. (Later, I learned

HMO doctors are inclined to first try less expensive approaches. In my case eight critical months slipped by before the referral was made.)

The sonogram revealed a large tumor on the left ovary and the uterus, plus two CA-125 tumor markers were elevated. Thus, when I underwent a hysterectomy and exploratory surgery on June 17, 1992, no big surprises were forthcoming. Cancer deaths tended to run in my family.

It was late-stage ovarian/endometrial cancer — Stage IIIC that had metastasized throughout the peritoneal cavity and also to one or two lymph nodes (the doctors weren't sure about the second). Naively, I thought that if enough poisonous chemicals were poured into me there was a good chance for recovery. Although my spirits were buoyed by the high optimism of the very caring doctors and nurses, the three courses of intense chemotherapy I endured did fail. On June 30, 1994 I was told that further toxigenic treatments would be counter productive as my "immune system couldn't be pounded anymore." Prognosis: Terminal. I now fully comprehended why this form of cancer was called *the silent killer* and my world shriveled. But when my husband reminded me that we had successfully tackled other seemingly intractable health problems using natural approaches, we both took the cue and spun into action.

Frantic research and determined efforts initiated in part by a nearby nutrition specialist and naturopathic physician, and approved and monitored by my oncologist, internist, and gynecologist, as well as other specialists, first only brought uncertain improvement; but presently, remission seems possible. During these years I experienced seven surgeries plus other critical events, three of which are described: one surgery to free up my intestines damaged by the chemotherapy; another to remove a four-centimeter brain tumor (possibly metastatic); and emergency treatment to dissolve highly dangerous blood-clot parts that had migrated to my lungs (again, caused by past chemotherapy). Today I am left with a damaged digestive system requiring the systematic intake of digestive enzymes; a damaged vascular system requiring a measured intake of warfarin (rat poison) to thin the blood and thus prevent clotting; and chronic anemia which is hard to treat and brings with it chronic fatigue. As well, my bones and teeth appear weakened. The chemotherapy has also left me with head tremors which, while commonly mild, can be an impediment.

When non-toxic patented drugs are unavailable for a specific application such as battling cachexia or restoring a chemo-damaged immune system, less powerful, bio-active nutritional substances are brought into play. Because such substances can serve a specific function not unlike that of the more benign patented prescription drugs (when available), they are spoken of as *nutraceuticals*. My doctors, especially the naturopathic physician, also explained matters this way: When the body is invaded, it means the malignancy has overcome the immune defenses either by stealth (mimicking normal cells) or by overpowering a weakened system. Everyone in his lifetime gets cancer, but most immune systems function as Providence intended and the errant cells are consumed. Chemotherapy, by contrast, poisons both good and bad cells and it becomes a race of sorts. Sometimes the patient does win, but often it's the malignancy. In losing, the hapless cancer victim is now faced with a double-barreled problem: a greatly damaged system resulting in implacable cachexia plus surviving cancer cells made that much more resistant. Thus, any effort to rehabilitate the weakened immune system, let alone defeat the more virulent cancer cells, becomes all the more problematic. This is where I stood as my compromised immune system had to be enhanced beyond the pre-chemo level and malignant cells starved (anti-angiogenesis) and perhaps rendered recognizable systemically. Nontoxic, bio-active nutraceuticals occurring naturally are unlike something like warfarin rat poison simply repackaged (e.g., Coumadin).

Tuesday, July 12, 1994 actually presaged a near miss, because the subsequent observation of numerous terminal cases keenly demonstrated that had I started my rehabilitation even a week or two later, I would not have made it. And I started my course just 12 days after being told *officially* that all had failed and I had no realistic hope of survival. My case had so many near misses, in fact, that I am not only amazed but truly thankful. But fighting such an uphill battle is not easy and often fosters acute anxiety. Observation: many, if not most terminal or near-terminal cancer victims would rather face death than deal with this kind of uncertainty. I need to add that just because something worked for me, it does not mean it will work for someone else. Also, I had made up my mind to simply treat my ovarian cancer as a chronic disease as virtually no hope existed for a complete cure. This, too, would be difficult for some people to accept.

Now, to my substantive rehabilitation effort. Because of my desperate condition, my husband and I knew that we only had one chance and that it had to hit the target. Thus a shotgun approach was used and the *shot* consisted of the following: very large dosages of a gently processed and clinically tested shark cartilage (BeneFin brand); some bovine cartilage; initially, Essiac tea alternated with a Hoxsey-like formula; pancreatic and digestive enzymes; acidophilus; and a variety of antioxidants and immune boosters, including vitamins E and C plus selenium and beta carotene along with CoQ1O, oriental mushrooms, flaxseed oil, cat's claw, grape seed extract, soy products, garlic and more recently MGN-3. One of the Biblical foods, apricot kernels, had become a part of the regimen until recently when it was forced off the market. For a time it appeared that a similar Government edict might snare the critical anti-angiogenic shark cartilage I am taking, as well as MGN-3. But in this case, countervailing forces prevailed and I got to live. To be sure, the influence of the highly profitable pharma-medical industry is considerable and there is no shortage of Government corruption. (A new wrinkle — powerful special interests have started to wine and dine judges!)

"Nothing should be considered ancillary." Thus, targeted physical and deep fresh-air breathing exercises; meditation; guided imagery; hypnotic sessions; avoidance of carcinogens; ingestion of organic foods, preferably home grown; attention to support mechanisms and the avoidance of stress were enumerated by my attending doctors (especially the oncologist and naturopathic physician) as essential aspects of my rehabilitation program. This is the explanation given: Just the opposite of the weight of the preverbal straw, these modalities, synergistically or otherwise, might provide just the lift necessary for a favorable outcome. I was encouraged to attend weekly GYN support sessions at the Cancer Care Center in Tucson, which I have since 1995 with near-perfect attendance. Similarly, since 1995 my husband and I attended all of the annual three-day Cancer Control Society conventions held outside of Los Angeles.

For nearly ten years now my natural strategy has kept me alive. Incredibly, my CA-125 recently dropped to 4 and the nurses surrounded me in open astonishment, as did my oncologist. The doctor had me stay after the examination to discuss plans to include some complementary modalities in his practice. Accordingly, days later his short impromptu visit to the woman's support group to which I belong was warmly received, as he was the first and only doctor to sit in and visit since its inception in 1994! This illustrates why I have to give much credit to my doctors and the fine support personnel. Careful selection pays!

Next, I have to give key credit to the taking of huge doses of premium grade shark cartilage. Since my long-standing rheumatoid arthritis symptoms all but disappeared within 10 days of its start, I knew even at this very early stage that the cartilage was likely doing something. Similarly, a *bouncy* pattern traced by the string of later CA-125 results was distinctly associated with cartilage intake. I found the dosages had to be maintained. The last eight very low markers suggest that I have gone into a remission of sorts, rather than the usual control mode wherein tiny tumors remain active yet unable to grow or metastasize. This is due most likely to the anti-angiogenic power to starve tumors that researchers found in the gently processed cartilage I get from Lane Labs-USA, Inc. {www.lanelabs.com}. It should be stressed that harshly processed cartilage purchased on the open market has been shown not to have the same level of power.

It is difficult to express the shock I experienced when in April of 2000 I ran out of the digestive enzymes I first took in July of 1994 (soon adding acidophilus, and just 19 months later, more enzymes). In that period, my chemo-damaged digestive tract had nearly caused my death and now the damage remains as I faced starvation anew. The beneficial effects of the enzymes had come on gradually, but the recent interruption caused an explosive return of the original upsets. Urgently, the enzyme supply was replenished and the digestive upsets quickly subsided. Similarly, when I stopped taking the shark cartilage or lowered the dosage significantly, the cancer symptoms returned and/or I had an ominous rise in the CA-125. When I returned to the high cartilage dosages, a favorable response also came quickly. (But in the beginning, it took 20 weeks before it appeared that this cartilage protocol had indeed started to control my cancer.) It needs to be stressed that my immune-boosting program largely was professionally tailored using extensive blood tests — two of which involved 10 vials each.

GEORGE TAYLOR
MALIGNANT MELANOMA

Sometime prior to 1980, I was diagnosed with malignant melanoma on the upper left part of my chest. This was surgically removed at the VA Hospital in Dallas, Texas, with no further complications for about 12 years.

Around 1989, I was again diagnosed with malignant melanoma, this time it was on my lower-left back. This was surgically removed at M.D. Anderson Cancer Center in Houston, Texas.

Initially, it appeared that both the above surgeries were successful. However, as it turns out, that was not the case. In December 1992, I discovered a small lump, about the size of a grape, located in a lymph node in my left armpit. This discovery had ominous and deadly implications. Apparently one of the previous melanomas was still with me and had started to spread, and spreading melanoma is usually a death sentence. My oncologist informed me that I probably had less than three months to live. I was 68 years old at the time.

Appointments were made to start conventional treatment. However, sometime after my first surgery in 1980, I had attended a lecture given by Charlotte Gerson about a cancer therapy developed by her father, Dr. Max Gerson. After reviewing the Gerson literature and talking to a *terminal* cancer patient that had been healed by the Gerson Therapy eleven years earlier, I decided I would first go to the Gerson clinic in Mexico and get another perspective.

Melanoma kills quickly and time was of the essence. In less than two weeks after I discovered the tumor, I was at the Gerson Clinic in Tijuana, Mexico. The tumor was rapidly increasing in size. It had grown to about the size of a tennis ball and was starting to interfere with the circulation in my left arm, resulting, at times, in numbness. The discomfort and minor pain involved was starting to interfere with my sleep.

The Gerson doctor indicated that with melanoma, the therapy, if successful, would either 1) kill the tumor, and the necrotic tissue would then be excreted during the course of the therapy's very intense detoxification program, or 2) the tumor would become encapsulated and then be removed by surgery at the end of the therapy. The therapy was said to last at least two years and sometimes longer.

During my three and a half weeks at the clinic I became convinced that my best chance of survival was to continue with the Gerson Therapy. Once home, I informed my oncologist of this decision. Against his advice, and with the exception of blood tests every six weeks, all other plans having to do with conventional treatment were canceled.

I immediately started the rigorous schedule required by the therapy, which included, among many other things: 13 organic juices a day, five coffee-retention enemas a day, frequent castor oil treatments, and blood tests every six weeks. With minor modifications, this intense, time-consuming (12 to 14 hours a day) schedule continued until the therapy was completed.

After the first year of therapy I was starting to feel really great. My energy levels were relatively high and (foolishly) I decided to ratchet my exercise routine up a notch, from walking to running. Unknown to me, the extra energy needed for strenuous exercise was being taken away from the energy reserves needed by my immune system to heal the cancer. This negative development was indicated on December 16, 1993 when the first CAT scan was done; it showed the tumor was growing and starting to divide into two separate tumors. Otherwise the scan was *negative for disease.* In looking back on this incident, I think the therapy was temporarily reversed (by me) from overdoing my exercise program.

The above incident was worrisome, so I returned to the Gerson Clinic for one week. While there, I received Laetrile injections to increase the tumor's sensitivity to heat, concurrently with hydrotherapy (in the form of extremely hot baths) — it seems that cancer cells die at 104+ degrees. By the end of the week there was a dramatic and unmistakable reduction in the size of the tumor.

In December 1994, at 70 years of age, I finally completed the therapy. During the past year there had been a modest increase in the size of the tumor and it had become almost rock hard. We assumed the tumor was now encapsulated, and arrangements were made to have it removed. As a retired Navy man, I decided to have the surgery performed at a military hospital. Wilford Hall Medical Center (WHMC), Lackland Air Force Base, Texas, near San Antonio, was chosen.

The Gerson doctor requested a "conservative lumpectomy procedure" be performed on a "stage III left-axillary-metastasized superficial spreading malignant melanoma" tumor and advised against "lymphatic dissection or wider excision unless surgical margins are demonstrably infiltrated."

However, the military doctors did not agree. They were certain that wider excisions would be required. They assured me they would encounter black cancerous areas throughout this part of my body, particularly in the lymph system, and these would have to be removed. We finally agreed that they would conform to the Gerson protocols and remove absolutely nothing unless it was "demonstrably infiltrated."

It should be mentioned, that WHMC Doctors and staff were outstanding throughout this. It was obvious they had not encountered anything like this before, and there was considerable interest in how it would turn out. I found the military doctors to be relatively open-minded, (as compared to the civilian medical establishment), which was gratifying indeed. That having been said, it should be added that they were more than a little bewildered by my chosen *therapy*. My oldest son remembers hearing one doctor refer to the Gerson Therapy as "something out of the Twilight Zone."

WHMC is a teaching hospital and the Commanding Officer/Chief Surgeon was in charge at my surgery. Later, after the tumor was removed, he told me there had been a number of other surgeons in the operating room to observe the procedure. It was his opinion that, collectively, among those present, they had probably performed hundreds of lumpectomies, but none had ever seen a tumor that looked like the one that had just been removed.

He said the tumor was indeed encapsulated. It was encased in about 1/4" to 3/4" of scar tissue, just like the scar tissue you might see from a healed cut on a person's body. He stated that wide excisions were not required and that the surgical margins were *clean*, including the surface area of the scar tissue. He informed me that the survival rate for this type of cancer is less than 1% and that I was very lucky to be alive. It was his opinion that the Gerson therapy had done exactly what they said it would do.

In the later written tissue report from the Pathology Lab, the tumor was described as an "unoriented mass 9.0 x 8.0 x 4.5 cm [3.5" x 3.2" x 1.77"], red, firm, and nodular." As for the diagnosis, "These findings are most consistent with the diagnosis of malignant melanoma."

Since the removal of the tumor, two additional CAT scans have been done (July 1995 and February 1996) with no areas of concern indicated.

On 23 March, 1998, a complete follow-up exam for malignant melanoma was performed by Major John G. LeVasseur, Staff Dermatologist, Keesler Medical Center, Keesler Air Force Base, Bioxi, Mississippi, with "no significant laboratory abnormalities noted."

In closing, seven years and three months after being declared *terminal*, I continue to follow (by choice) my own modified version of the Gerson protocols.

As of this writing I am 76 years old. I enjoy buoyant health, which is an understatement, for sure. My energy levels are high, and I am very active. Among many other things, as part of my normal exercise practice, I will walk or jog (or both) 3 miles, usually every other day. When I choose to do so, which is not very often (I believe it's called laziness), I can do three ten minute miles and complete the run in 30 minutes.

My health is such that I can pursue various career options if I wish. I am free to go back into any of the ocean related professions with which I am familiar, including Commercial Diving, salvage and underwater demolition. However, I have really come to appreciate this game called *semi-retirement,* and I will probably just leave it alone for now. In any event, it is truly a nice thing, at the age of 76, to be able to make choices which are in no way influenced by concerns about ill health.

Since 1992, cancer has been an incomparable teacher. One of the many things this adventure has taught me is that while the 'clock' (of aging) cannot be stopped, it can be rolled back and slowed down. In the process of learning from these experiences, I have come to believe that rapid aging and most degenerative diseases (including cancer) are caused by a progressive poisoning of the body, which can be reversed.

By most estimates, my health at this point in time is probably as good as it was in my early 50s and, in many ways, even better. To see me is to believe it!

Barring accident, I continue to look forward to a long, healthy, very active, and productive life.

JOHN E. PETERS
NON-SMALL CELL LUNG CANCER

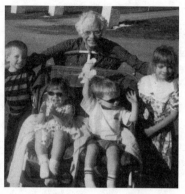

I refused a biopsy and had open-chest surgery where the tumor was obtained, sectioned, slides made and diagnosed by a pathologist.

X-rays and CAT scans showed a tumor a little larger than a golf ball in my right lung. The doctors were 90% sure from x-rays and CAT scans that it was cancer, and the diagnosis was made after the surgery, since I had refused a biopsy (because it might cause the cancer to spread). During the surgery, they discovered the cancer had already spread and they could not get it all. Thus, I underwent about 23 radiation treatments. The cancer had not caused much pain, but I was coughing a lot, before and after the surgery. The radiation treatments did not bother me at first, but became devastating at the end. I still have radiation fibrosis from the radiation.

I continued my life as normal as possible. I only missed four weeks of work from the surgery and only a few days from radiation treatments. As a scientist with excellent access to both allopathic and alternative methods, I carefully researched lung cancer and called the only long term survivor I could locate.

About a year after the surgery my cough got worse and I became very weak, sick and lost almost 50 pounds.

Nothing the doctors could do helped and they again wanted to do a biopsy. Again, I refused, but I did have a video bronchoscopic examination. I was told that the cancer was definitely back, and that I had to have surgery and radiation again, and this time I would also have to have chemotherapy. The doctors did not tell me that the five year survival rate was essentially zero and their treatments would dramatically reduce the quality of my life, even if I survived the treatments.

When I refused all treatment, the doctors were upset, argued with me, and said that I was committing suicide. I told them that they had almost killed me the first time with radiation and surgery, and there was no way I would submit to that type of therapy again, especially chemotherapy. I told them that I might die, but it would not be at their hands. Needless to say, I severed all relations with the oncologists.

Knowing the five-year survival rate was essentially zero, I had fully accepted that I would die and realized it was up to God as to when I die. Thus, I prayed for divine guidance and vowed to do everything I could do to follow His guidance completely. Then I was able to quit worrying about death and devote all my efforts to finding out what I was to do and then doing it faithfully. I know that God helps those who help themselves, and when we have diligently done everything we can do, God does the rest and miracles occur. The Bible says "pray without ceasing," and in my situation I believe it also meant to work without ceasing while trusting God completely with the outcome, as the Gerson therapy, which I believed offered me my best chance of surviving, was labor intensive.

The Gerson Institute did suggest a two week stay in their hospital to learn the procedure, so I bought airline tickets to San Diego, California where someone from the Institute would meet me and take me to the CHIPSA Hospital. Unfortunately, they could not accept me for about six weeks. Since I was still losing weight and getting progressively weaker, I could not afford to wait six weeks. Thus, I began doing the Gerson therapy at home.

Since I could not find anyone nearby who had experience with the therapy, I had to rely mostly on Dr. Gerson's book, *A Cancer Therapy: Results of Fifty Cases.* Contacts at CHIPSA were very helpful and sent me everything I needed to do the therapy at home. At first, I was overwhelmed by the tremendous amount of work and discipline required. Without my vow to God to do everything possible to follow the therapy, I'm sure that even with lots of help and support from loyal friends, the Gerson Institute and CHIPSA, I would not have done the full therapy — coffee enemas and all. But thank God I did. In only three weeks, I had gained six pounds and was feeling better. Thus, when the Gerson Institute called to let me know I could come to the hospital, I told them I was doing the therapy at home, it was working, and I no longer needed to be admitted to their hospital.

For several months, the Gerson therapy was the center of my life. Then I was able to go back to work part-time and then full-time, while still on the full therapy. I would make five 8 ounce juices at one time in the morning, another four 8 ounce juices at noon, and four more after work. I continued this for about 18 months and carried a quart thermos full of cold juice everywhere I went. Then I began to cut back on the juices and went off the full therapy. Today I still don't consume animal products (except a small amount of fish occasionally) and drink about four glasses of juice a day.

Without the Gerson therapy I would have been dead a long time ago and would never have known any of my five grandchildren. Words cannot express my gratitude to the Gerson Institute and to my wonderful supportive friends who have helped me constantly for the past 12 years.

The most important part in my healing from metastasized lung cancer was my accepting that I was going to die, praying for divine guidance and doing everything that I could do to find God's plan for me and then following it to the best of my ability. When I did all that I could do, God did the rest. Thirteen years later there is no sign of cancer. Thus, I am glad to share my experience with those who wish to contact me.

CORY HOWARD
BREAST CANCER

In July of 1996 they found a tumor. I tried to get rid of it with Chinese medicine and proteolytic enzymes to no avail. For my temporary peace of mind I had surgery in Sept. 1997. The diagnosis is what I thought it was — breast cancer. I was paralyzed with fear. I visited the Women's Cancer Resource Center in Minneapolis where I was living at the time. The director, whose name escapes me now, said the one single thing that seemed to save my life at the moment, "...you have time to make the right decision for yourself." Suddenly, I could breathe again. I spent the next few months researching and reading books about what was going on inside my body. I also started praying like a maniac. I have always been a very curious person and a hungry searching person in terms of spiritual development. I knew this was a call of some sort, but I couldn't figure out what it was because there was so much emotional debris flying around inside me. My partner of 4 years decided that he was unable to hang in there with me. This was actually a blessing in disguise, but very painful at the time. My cat and companion of 19 years also died within two months of my diagnosis of cancer. I had already started weaning myself from my business that was really in need of me moving on. So a lot was happening all at once for me. A call to start finding a way back to myself.

I spent the following year in one big long nervous breakdown, trying to hold on to some pieces of my sanity and dignity while trying to figure out how I was going to save my life.

I have always been a part of the *alternative* community, so finding healers and alternative medicine people was not difficult, but back then there was little support for that sort of thing. My family was terrified. We had all watched on as my Mom died of this illness years before, and now here I was 39, with cancer! What?! When I was nine I had a series of dreams about having cancer. I knew somewhere inside that this was coming down the pike for me. This is not some twisted new age notion of creating ones own reality either. Anyway, I hooked myself up with a naturopath in St. Paul who helped me develop a protocol of supplements. I worked with a Chinese MD who was wonderful, doing acupuncture to keep my head and heart relatively straight and to boost immunity. I worked with a chiropractor who did energy medicine similar to Qigong. I even worked with an extraordinary Native woman participating in healing ceremonies. My diet was always pretty clean. I was just stressed out *all* the time, anxious *all* the time. Talk about exhausting. A year after the first surgery I decided to move back to the east coast, Pennsylvania, where I was from. I wanted to be nearer to my family and to move on from life in Minnesota, where I had lived for 21 years. All the doors were closing and it didn't take a rocket scientist to see this. So I moved.

I also want to mention that, within the first week or two of the first diagnosis, I heard several voices in my head. One said, "What you believe in will heal you." The other said, "This is the last fear." Both are gifts to me that I treasure to this day as information from a deeper source about the truth of my illness. I realized that breast cancer is about nurturance, self-nurturance. Women do amazing acts of giving in the world, but we aren't always very adept at providing that same giving to ourselves. I also think cancer is about love and the lack of it or the active pushing away of it — as in my case! So the call for me was beginning to have a definition, love yourself and hold your love high.

Over the next two years, I developed tumors again, right next to the previous tumor, three in all. I always continued my aggressive supplement protocol and herbs and various other healing techniques - Reiki, Qigong, body work, and therapy of all types. I was bound to exorcise this thing without killing myself in the process. Traditional treatment was never a real option for me. Too scary, too cruel. (I received a certified letter from my first set of doctors, two women, telling me how disappointed they were in me — how healing!) I just kept sprouting a new tumor every spring; I kept having them out. One of the times, I had some lymph nodes taken out too, because they were swollen, and I was anxious. I don't recommend this though. The only reason to take lymph nodes is to know how much chemo to give and to stage you. Both points are non-issues to me. I still suffer from the violence done to the soft delicate tissue of my armpit.

When I found my latest tumor (and there is a lot of story between all the tumors in terms of my personal development, people met, protocols tried...), tumor #4, I became despondent. I have tried everything that I know but have found no relief form this. How do I get off this train anyway? I fell into a depression and stopped pretty much everything. I was not employed and had very little support. I floated for months and months. I wanted to die, or I thought I wanted to die. I was pooped and lonely and alone. I couldn't find anything else inside to keep me going. I didn't have work. I don't have kids. What could I wrap my life around that gave it meaning? I couldn't find anything.

I had a friend I met who also has cancer — lymphoma. He would give me pep talks periodically, enough to keep me going. Slowly I pulled myself out, by the grace of Spirit. Also, I had hooked up with a group of amazingly smart women on a listserv on the Internet that all deal with their cancer alternatively. I would get great info and support from them. About the time I was pulling out of the funk, I discovered that I had 12 small tumors in my lungs, along with a large primary tumor in what is left of my breast tissue. So this is my challenge now. With this discovery I realized it was time to go to a clinic.

I chose Humlegaarden in Denmark. My friends sent me the money, after a fund-raising letter I had written. While I was there (March 2002), a lot of things happened. Most moving to me was having my heart open up and realize that the other part of the calling to me was from Spirit to receive all the healing that everyone all around me everyday, every minute is sending to me. I can tell you that it is a whole lot easier to give than to receive, to really take in. I realized that the heart is the doorway to all healing. Maybe everyone knows this and I guess I did too, but I couldn't quite get into my heart, she was so closed off. My loneliness was my own. My sorrow was my own. I realized that everything I have needed has been right with me all along. So I am having a renaissance of faith. I am not alone; never was, no matter what I felt or thought. I know now that all the pills I take and food I eat and prayers I say will be hyper-super powered now because they come from a deep place in me, from a loving place inside me and they go out to a loving Spirit that is with me, in me all the time. No matter what happens, I am going to be okay. I know it sounds weird or pollyanna, but I know in my heart it is true. I have good days and not so good days with this whole thing. It's my humanity I am retrieving with all the love and tenderness I can afford myself at any given moment.

My protocol is like this — and I take a lot of it right now:

I take Proboost, thymic protein

RM 10, Garden of Life product (I think these guys are good, my opinion only.)

CoQ10

Vascustatin and AAG herb (anti-angiogenesis herb, bindweed)

Ai/e 10, a colostrum product developed by Dr. Jesse Stoff

High doses of Selenium and E

Enzymes of all sorts

Pure Synergy, a green food

Pau d'arco

I inject 14 different homeopathics I received from Denmark every evening (It's not as tough as you might think; trust me, if I can do it, anyone can.)

I take a good multi-vitamin designed for women by Pure

Synergy

I take melatonin at night

LDN — low-dose naltrexone raises the endorphin levels in the body (Bernard Bihari's research — also one of my doctors)

Natural progesterone cream, a la Dr. John Lee and David Zava's work.

When I have my stuff together in one place, I also juice every morning.

I get monthly colonics along with lymphatic massage and spend time in a far-infared sauna.

I am constantly researching other things to do everyday.

There is a lot I didn't put in, specifics that might be more helpful than my philosophizing, so you are welcome to contact me. It's been an extraordinary trip. As I write this today, I feel heavy and weary; but I still feel basically good and strong. Cancer is a tricky bastard and I know this. I work very hard at staying humble and present everyday so that I can enjoy what is here for me. This week I lost two friends to cancer — brave, courageous, lovely women. So I'm pissed, but still willing to be here with God, Spirit. There is too much else I want to do! I'm just getting started.

I wholly and completely support alternative approaches to cancer treatment. I also support each person's need to follow their own path. We are all delivered an incredible bill of goods here on Earth, and whatever I can do to help facilitate that in this life, hallelujah.

I believe what was most effective in my healing was my commitment to myself. Finding something bigger than me to help me along.

Finding enough support to keep going when my faith fails me.

My tenacious spirit and a complete unwillingness to die, at this moment.

Doing everything possible to support my immune system.

Educating myself.

Eating well.

Letting go of as much stress as possible — *It really isn't worth it!*

Letting go of the fear and rage — to the best of my ability each day.

Be human, expressing my natural loving kindness.

PRAYING — dialogue with Spirit.

FRED ROBERTSON
PROSTATE CANCER

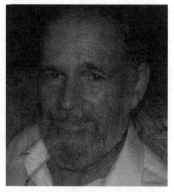

I know that having a devoted spiritual life and a positive attitude was a must for me. We all need to be in a better frame of mind when we are told disturbing news. The positive side has been my life. The spiritual path I have chosen gave me the ultimate experience of my life. My Spirit has soared to a point in meditation beyond imagination. To have been that great is beautiful. If only all could.

I know that Essiac is the main reason that I have felt so good for the past 6 years. Not only have I reached remission, but I have a life better today than throughout my life. My oncologist told me after the 16 months on Essiac treatment that I was in remission from a rare blood disorder that I had needed monthly treatments for since 1973. Can it be anything else? Doubtful.

I am very fortunate to be able to tell the story of my survival for all to read. I know that *all* of these were needed for me. My life today is great to say the least and I am prepared for what is to be...

He has always had a plan for me as with all of us.

God Bless in Master's name.

Please contact me if I can help in any way.

DR. REGINA L. CHORSKY
BREAST CANCER

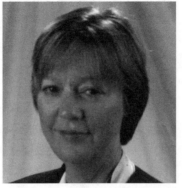

In November, 2000, I had a biopsy performed on what I thought was a benign fibroadenoma. Nine years previously I had a benign fibroadenoma removed from my left breast. I am a pathologist, so I was pretty confident that it was benign on palpation. I looked at the slides myself and couldn't make the call on it, so I sent the slides to another pathologist who was a friend. Just before Thanksgiving day my friend called me with the bad news that it was "Invasive ductal carcinoma." The mass was 3 cm and there were 4 positive lymph nodes out of twenty. There was some skin involvement, to the surprise of myself, two oncology surgeons and a hematology oncologist, because of its benign appearance.

All in all, I wasn't happy about the prognosis. I began doing things on faith and following my instincts. Even though by my standards as a pathologist my future looked grim, I decided to do what I wanted. I didn't want chemo or radiation, but did choose the surgery. Immediately after the reduction in tumor load by surgery, I began to feel better and have more energy. I started taking half a bottle of fermented soy (Haelan 951) a day. It smelled and tasted terrible. I continued to feel better, have more energy, sleep and eat better. Through out this time my faith in God and myself deepened. Now I feel stronger emotionally, physically and spiritually than I ever have before. The best advice I can offer anyone in this situation is to pray about it, ask God for guidance and follow your heart. I believe you will know the best approach to take to become well again.

The most meaningful and effective part of my healing has been a deeper relationship with God.

HELEN CURRAN
MALIGNANT MELANOMA

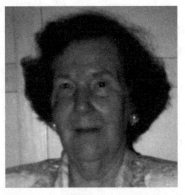

I had a brown mole on my face ever since I was a teenager. I blame it on the fact that when I was a child, I used to try very hard to get a tan, but since I had red hair and freckles, the only thing I succeeded in doing was getting one sunburn after another. By the time I was 55, the mole had turned black and my cheek was puffy. I was afraid to go to the doctor, but eventually I was more afraid not to.

The mole was taken off my cheek in my surgeon's office, and it was very deep. The diagnosis from the biopsy was malignant melanoma. I went into the hospital for what was called a "wide excision," which left me with a round scar on my face about the size of a fifty-cent piece. I was surprised that no lymph nodes were removed. Because the technician had sounded evasive to me when I had the liver scan, I asked my surgeon if the cancer had metastasized to my liver. My husband was in the room when I asked and the surgeon replied, "No." There is no polite way of saying that this was a lie, whether to protect my feelings or his or both, I cannot say. This took place in January of 1978.

I became progressively weaker and my family doctor recommended that I go to a world-famous cancer clinic in Los Angeles, where they did various tests and recommended that I have my jugular vein removed to keep the cancer from spreading. I was, of course, frightened and asked them to check with my surgeon, who told them the situation. They relayed the news that I had a few months to live to me over the telephone. They said there was nothing they could do for melanoma that has metastasized. I was alone at home and I paced through the house like a mad woman. Then I phoned my surgeon, and he admitted he had not told me the truth. I was panic stricken and my husband was devastated.

In the meantime, my best friend Laura had surgery for ovarian cancer and refused the chemotherapy that was strongly recommended to her. She found (through an acquaintance of her daughter) an American chiropractor who did metabolic therapy for cancer patients in a Mexican hospital. At the time, he rented bedspace in a Mexican hospital. He now has a clinic of his own, but because of the situation in California, I don't think he would want his name published. Laura had been in Mexico for one week on the dismal afternoon I was given a death sentence, and I phoned her there. She tried to persuade me to join her, but I had been well indoctrinated. I told her I thought what she was doing was quackery, and if it worked, surely the American doctors would be using it. I had an awful lot to learn in those days.

A few days later my family doctor recommended a CAT scan of my liver followed by a sonogram. The two tumors on my liver were still there. I was scarcely able to walk by this time, and I had very little appetite. I finally decided to join Laura in Tijuana. At least I would be with people like myself and not feel so alone. My husband agreed and on Sunday, March 12, 1978, we took the two-hour drive from Laguna Beach to Tijuana. The doctor was waiting for me at the hospital, and I asked him if he could cure liver cancer. He said the three best words I ever expect to hear: "Livers are easy." My husband and I looked at each other, and I'm sure my thoughts were his. Either this was one of the quacks we had been warned against, or else this tall man with the booming voice was a miracle worker. Since this took place almost eleven years ago, I think you know how we feel about him today.

I was given three hours of drips containing 15 grams of Laetrile, 25 grams of Vitamin C, and some Vitamin B. Since I have allergies, I lay in bed stiff with fear for about ten minutes expecting who-knows-what to happen — maybe the famous cyanide poisoning we hear so much about but never see. A plate of raw fruits and vegetables were brought in for my supper and I picked at this with my one free hand. I finally fell asleep repeating to myself, "Livers are easy."

I have had many people say to me that it was my faith in my therapy that cured me. This is not so, at least in the beginning. I went to Tijuana thinking I was turning to quackery although hoping by some miracle I was not. In two days I felt considerably better. My appetite was back. The gas pains were almost gone thanks to the enzymes I took with each meal. And when my husband came to visit me after only those two days, I was able to take a walk with him to a park about one-quarter of a mile away. I knew I was going to live, and I knew who the quacks were now.

I stayed in Tijuana for two weeks. My therapy consisted of large amounts of supplements, coffee enemas, and various homeopathic drops. Also, I had a daily injection of a formula made from my own blood. Today I understand that my doctor has added several new components to the therapy.

I had checkups every two weeks when I returned home. After a few months these were cut back to once a month and then every six weeks. After a year and a half, I had another liver scan and was overjoyed to learn that the tumors were gone. Two years ago I had a sebaceous cyst removed from my head and I was pleased that after I told my surgeon where I had gone for therapy, he said, "You can't quarrel with success, Helen." These eleven years have been the happiest of my married life. You never take life for granted again, but I feel certain if I stick to the diet and take my Laetrile, I will probably outlive most of the people I know.

I believe there is no magic bullet. Laetrile is very important, but so is diet as well as the supplement regimen, the coffee enemas, support from one's family, guided imagining, a loving doctor, homeopathy, avoidance of toxins — and here you must read and learn. It has now been 25 years since I was told I had two to three months to live. My doctor is no longer alive. I loved him dearly, and the last thing he said to me on the phone before he died was, "Good-bye. I love you." I get to the Cancer Control Society's Convention every year and usually give my testimonial and get a big hand. Many of the doctors there give me a hug and a kiss. I guess I'm sort of a symbol of what can be done. I'm on a list of people you can phone if you've been told there is nothing you can do (www.brave-souls.com). I've written a book, which is selling pretty well, called *APRICOT POWER: How Laetrile Cured My Cancer*. I also run a holistic club in Leisure World, where I bring only holistic doctors to speak once a month.

PATRICIA GULER
BREAST CANCER

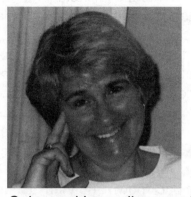

I am Patricia A. Guler, and I was diagnosed with breast cancer in June, 1994 at 48 years of age. I was living in Connecticut at the time. The surgeon who did the biopsy and made recommendations about subsequent treatment for my cancer was a teaching surgeon at University of Connecticut and very well respected. He wanted to remove a quarter of my left breast, all my lymph nodes and to give me radiation followed by chemo. At the time I was extremely fatigued and had bronchitis that six different prescriptions wouldn't clear up, so a respiratory specialist put me on a breathing apparatus and told me I'd have bronchitis the rest of my life. I cut my finger on Mothers Day and it still hadn't healed by June 7th. There were also other little things that were just not right with my body. I asked myself how I was going to go through all this treatment in the condition I was in.

My parents who are interested in alternative medicine called me from Minnesota and begged me to go to Dr. W. Douglas Brodie in Reno, Nevada. I called Dr. Brodie and he recommended I come out there and at least have my immune system checked before I started with all of this. Four days later I was in his office, pathology report from the biopsy at Hartford Hospital in hand, having a blood test called a darkfield. From this he could evaluate that my immune system was working at twenty percent of its overall capacity with the white cells, the infection fighters, working at only five percent. No wonder I couldn't fight off bronchitis and heal cuts. I stayed out in Reno for three weeks taking IV's for my immune system that also included laetrile. Each Monday we would do another darkfield test and you could see on the television monitor how much more aggressive the white cells were. The second week I was there, Dr. Brodie had a consultation with me and I remember him starting out by saying to me, "Pat, you're going to be just fine. When you get back to Connecticut, don't let them take a quarter of the breast, just take the lump to the margins and DON'T let them take any of your lymph nodes. Radiation is going to run your immune system back down and there is not much evidence that chemo is going to do you any good." He also told me that we could do a AMAS blood test about two months after the surgery so we would know how the cancer was responding. I knew how good Dr. Brodies' credentials were and I trusted him.

When I went back to the motel that day I called my surgeon in Connecticut and told him that the surgery we had scheduled for two weeks later had to be done my way, or I would find another doctor. He agreed, but said I would have to sign a waiver as he would not be responsible. I agreed to sign it. When I got back to CT, I went in to my doctor for a pre-operative visit the day before surgery. He agreed to the surgery and lymph node part, but got very upset about no radiation or chemo. He stood up and as he was shaking his finger at me, he said: "That doctor doesn't know what he's talking about. You have a very aggressive cancer with an aneuploid stemline and you're going to be sorry, but you're not going to be here. You're going to be dead." It was unnerving, but I knew how I felt.

After the first week of treatment from Dr. Brodie I no longer was using the breathing apparatus, the cut on my finger healed as did my biopsy incision and I had an energy level I hadn't had in years. It was so nice to be feeling good again. I told him he agreed to do the surgery my way and I would sign whatever he needed me to sign. Three days after the surgery I had a post-operative visit with him. However I had obtained a copy of the post-op pathology report prior to this visit and part of it read "residual tumor, turned rubbery pink tissue, no carcinoma found."

When I was ready to leave the doctors examining room, he said to me: "Mrs. Smith (That was my last name at the time — I've since been widowed and remarried), occasionally I have a patient who chooses alternative treatment and I don't want to know today because I have a waiting room full of patients, but next time you come in I would like to know why you chose alternative treatment when insurance doesn't cover it?" Like my life isn't worth a plug nickel! It cost me around five thousand dollars for my treatment with Dr. Brodie back in 1994. I wrote my surgeon a two page letter explaining that three months after they found my cancer I had a daughter getting married. By the time of the wedding, I had made a lifestyle change in my eating habits (Dr. Brodie's diet) and looked better than I had in years. My treatment was painless. You sit in a recliner and take about a three hour drip and talk to the other patients. I learned a lot and I laughed a lot. I enjoyed the other patients; we all felt good about what we were doing to treat our cancer. Two months after the surgery, I had the AMAS blood test and it showed that I was cancer free. I still have all my lymph nodes, and never took radiation or chemo. As of today, I am almost eight years without any recurrence. I still go to Reno to have a check up with Dr. Brodie every couple of years. My mother sometimes goes with me, as she was his patient before I was and she is also eight years cancer free. I am convinced I would not have made it through all the conventional treatment they wanted to put me through with my immune system as weak as it was. I have often thanked Dr. Brodie for what I feel, for me, was a lifesaving treatment.

I believe the most important part of my healing was

keeping a positive attitude and having so much confidence in Dr. Brodie. Also, prayers gave me comfort and helped me accept God's Will.

I would be very happy to talk to anyone that has questions.

KEN WALKER
MULTIPLE MYELOMA

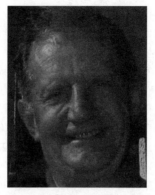

I am a Multiple Myeloma Cancer Survivor.

On March 19, 2001, and at the age of 67, my wife Deana and I were devastated by the news that I had only a short time to live. I was diagnosed as being in the latter stages of a rare form of bone marrow cancer, Multiple Myeloma.

My oncologist informed us there was no cure, only treatment — chemotherapy with all its dangerous side effects and Aredia infusions to strengthen and reduce bone pain. I chose to forego chemo, and take monthly infusions of Aredia. I also started on a very strict protocol I found through many hours of research to stop this cancer.

From the beginning, I believed in my heart of hearts that somewhere or somehow something could be done to conquer this adversary cancer. Or was this only wishful thinking? And why was God allowing me to die prematurely? Was there a purpose in this? Maybe so, because a lot of good has come out of this ordeal. Our family of 4 adult children and 7 grandchildren have been drawn closer together, and our many Christian friends have poured out their love and prayed that I would be given more years on this earth to be with my family and friends.

By May, I was in really bad shape. My oncologist told me

the "cancer was ravaging my bone marrow." My total protein was 12.3. My IGG serum was 7950. I had a monoclonal protein of 58.8 and 7.0 g/dl. I now had bone lesions in my head (holes in my skull), three broken ribs, cancer in my spine, and was unable to get up from a chair without help. I was trying to sleep sitting upright in a motorized recliner, taking both pain and sleeping pills. I was told I only had about 3 months to live.

It's now November 27, 2001. All of my cancer markers have fallen to just slightly above normal. My oncologist told me this past week that if I was coming in for a first time visit, they would not suspect cancer. He asked me to document what I had been doing to bring on such "fantastic results."

I spent hundreds of hours researching for a natural cure. I have documented everything I have taken. I have hundreds of pages of information. I have come to the conclusion that the following are the primary reasons I am where I am today. They are listed in the order of their importance to me.

1. My faith in a loving and merciful God. John 1:12 & Romans 10:9.

2. Poly-MVA - Dr. M. Garnett's creation which destroys cancer cells without the side effects. It is distributed by AMARC Inc.

3. MGN 3 - Triples natural killer cells. Created by a Pharmaceutical Company, in Tokyo.

4. Dr. Hulda Clark Ph.D. 21-day protocol.

NORMAN PIERSMA

MELANOMA

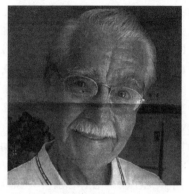

It all began in early October, 1990. Donna noticed blood on the back of my shirt. It turned out to be a mole that was bleeding, so I went to a skin cancer specialist for a diagnosis. I did not want him to do a biopsy. (My experience as a Veterinary Pathologist gave me a warning.) Since he convinced me that it was *not* melanoma, I let him go ahead. What I really wanted him to do was excise the area as did a Colombian surgeon did 20 years before with a melanoma site on my left shoulder. But the diagnosis *was* malignant melanoma stage III. The biopsy was taken 10/24/90.

On 10/30/90 they did extensive surgery on my back, removing skin the size of football. This was all in vain. On 4/01/91 we detected a lump in my right axillary region. On 4/09/91 the affected lymph node was removed and the path report was "metastatic melanoma." I was referred to Oncologist Raymond Lord of the Cancer Center in Kalamazoo, Michigan for an appointment on 4/30/91. He told me he had several cases like mine, but lost them all. I was told I was *terminal* with a maximum of six months to live. I rejected his protocol of chemos and never saw him again.

Instead I went to the Gerson clinic in Tijuana on 5/05/91. I started the Gerson Therapy ten minutes after arriving with

10 ounces of carrot juice. Since the Gerson Therapy is documented and well known, I'll not go into detail. We stayed only two weeks, long enough to learn all we needed to know for us to continue on this intense dietary regimen for the next year. Within three months, all palpable and visual evidence of the cancer had disappeared. I knew that I had beaten melanoma.

However, three years and three months later I detected another lymph node swelling in the same axillary site. On 8/29/94 I had it removed and again, the diagnosis was "metastatic melanoma." I then realized that I had gotten careless with my diet and lifestyle to the degree that melanoma returned. So back I went on a modified Gerson therapy using the new insights I had learned from the Hallelujah Diet. Instead of the difficult task of juicing greens, I took BarleyGreen. From that moment till now I have had perfect health. I learned my lesson. Practically all my nutrition is plant based, I drink pure water, and I get enough sunshine and exercise each day. I am the 5th fastest race walker in the nation in the age category 70 to 74. I'll be 75 next month.

"Most effective part of your healing?" Healing is never effected by an outside agent. Only the body is able to heal. All the body needs is two things: a thorough cleansing of excess toxins and waste products AND supplying the cells with all the nutrition it calls for. This is the formula for getting well and staying well. In these last ten years I've not had one sick day, have not taken one prescription, and have not once gone to a doctor because of illness.

BEATA BISHOP
MALIGNANT MELANOMA

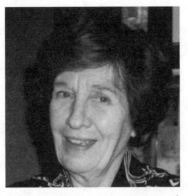

I underwent surgery to remove the tumor from my right shin. It was a wide excision, resulting in a large part of the flesh on my right leg being removed, and a skin graft effected, with skin from my left thigh. It was all enormously painful and disfiguring, and it took me some two months to be able to walk again. No other treatment was offered, only monthly and later six week check-ups. In December 1980, the consultant found a lump in my right groin and wanted to operate immediately to remove it, together with any lymph glands that were affected. By then I had done enough research to realize that this was a metastasis, and decided that further surgery would be useless, as the first operation had not solved the problem.

Naturally, I was shattered and in a state of shock, since the consultant had assured me that "he'd got it all" at the first go. So I refused surgery. By a wonderful coincidence, through a friend's friend, I heard about the Gerson Therapy.

I was lucky enough to find Dr. Gerson's granddaughter in London, which is where I live. After consulting her and reading Dr. Gerson's book, I decided to embark on this very demanding nutritional therapy, for the simple reason that it was logical and made sense. Its basic premise is that instead of concentrating on the removal or destruction of the tumor, which is only a symptom of an underlying general breakdown of the organism, the task is to detoxify the body and with the help of optimum nutrition bring the immune system to such a high level of efficiency that the body can heal itself.

In January 1981, I travelled to the Gerson clinic in Tijuana, Mexico, and stayed there for two months. Already, after 2 or 3 weeks, my early-stage diabetes mellitus disappeared, never to return; and my incipient osteoarthritis which had begun to distort the index and middle fingers of my right hand was also healed. After six weeks, my surgically mutilated right leg began to rebuild itself — new flesh appeared under the skin graft on the right side.

All this was enough to convince me that this therapy was working. I returned to London in March 1981 and continued with the intensive therapy until June 1982, gradually cutting down on it as instructed by my Mexican physician, and eventually coming off the therapy in March 1983.

It was a tough, monotonous and yet fascinating experience. The therapy consists of a vegetarian diet of organic vegetables and fruits (vegan for the first 6 weeks), with three square meals and 13 glasses of freshly made juice a day. There is also a range of medications (all natural substances), 5 coffee enemas a day for several months, then gradually diminishing in number, plus castor oil every other day, by mouth and enema. The diet excludes meat, eggs, cheese, salt, sugar, fats, alcohol, convenience foods and much more that is regarded as *normal* food. Since coming off the therapy I stick to the dietary rules, but occasionally add fish or organic chicken. I drink 2-3 glasses of juice a day and take half-strength coffee enemas every now and then. I am extremely fit and healthy, work hard and enjoy life.

The most important part of my healing was my total commitment to the Gerson therapy which was my choice, great curiosity to see if it could really work, and a strong wish to get well. I also had a wonderful support from my friends and my local doctor who was in favor of what I was doing.

I regarded this two years during which the therapy filled my life as an investment in a healthy future. It has certainly proved its worth.

THOMAS POWERS
MALIGNANT MELANOMA

I really didn't think I was a candidate for cancer. For the previous ten years I had watched my diet carefully, eating mostly organic foods and balanced meals and avoiding the candy, sodas, and other junk foods I had favored as a teenager. I was a non-smoker. I lived and worked in a rural setting in upstate New York, a remarkably unspoiled, unpolluted part of the world. I was forty-two, loved my work, had been happily married for four years, and had a two-year-old daughter plus three wonderful kids by a previous marriage — "everything to live for," as they say.

One day in March 1982, standing at the mirror shaving, I noticed a mole on my right temple. It wasn't very big, a little smaller than my little finger nail, and it didn't look particularly significant. Still, it hadn't been there before, so I mentioned it over the phone to my family physician. My description got an immediate response that I should have the mole removed and biopsied, right away. That surprised me somewhat, especially the sense of urgency. But no matter, I set up an appointment for April 22 at St. Francis Hospital in Lancaster, PA to get it taken off.

The surgeon who did the operation told me that most of these little "lumps and bumps" were benign, but if this one happened to turn out to be malignant, he would recommend further, more extensive surgery, followed by skin grafting. That was a little sobering, but I figured it was a standard pre-op speech, sort of like the life jacket instructions before a flight on a commercial airline, and let it go at that.

Eight days, later the lab report came back, and it was full of terms I couldn't understand, things like "compound nevus," "cellular unrest," "ballooning cytoplasmic change," "scattered mitoses," "junctional activity," and "Clark level 4," which would take on meaning only after I had been enlightened by the experts.

The bottom line of the report was clear enough, though: "malignant melanoma." I knew something about this form of cancer. Three friends of mine had died from melanoma, including one I had helped nurse during the final stages of his illness.

So, what next? Further surgery? Before I had time to consider my options very fully, the symptoms of the disease changed. Within a few days the melanoma returned to the operation site. And then dark brown growths began to appear on my chest and left arm. Now we had a different situation to address: melanoma with distant metastases. We consulted four different doctors, whose recommendations varied, but who agreed that neither surgery, radiation, nor any known form of chemotherapy, alone or in combination, offered hope for a cure of this type of cancer at this stage in its development. In unvarnished terms, my situation was viewed as terminal.

At this point, my family began to look for any resource outside the range of standard orthodox medicine that might offer hope of a cure. And at the third inquiry they hit the jackpot. The Gerson Institute in California reported that the Gerson therapy was highly successful as a treatment for this type of cancer. The fact that it had metastasized did not rule out the chances for success. The fact that I had not had radiation or chemotherapy was in my favor; it meant that my immune system had not been artificially suppressed and would respond better to this metabolic treatment plan — which was based on (1) drinking large amounts of freshly squeezed fruit and vegetable juices (thirteen eight-ounce glasses a day); (2) elimination of sodium, animal protein, and most fats from the diet; (3) supplementation with potassium salts, thyroid, Lugol solution, pancreatic enzymes, Niacin, and Vitamin B-12; and (4) detoxification by the use of coffee enemas.

On May 14, 1982, I began treatment on the Gerson therapy. To my, and my family's, eternal gratitude, it worked. By July 1, all visible tumors were gone. I had no further surgery. I had no chemotherapy or radiation. When my family physician saw me next, in September 1982, he was deeply impressed to find the disease in remission. I remained on the Gerson therapy for twenty months. I have had no recurrence of the cancer in the fourteen years since.

I have stayed in touch with the Gerson Institute over the years and have frequently recommended the Gerson therapy to other people with cancer. I personally know of a number of other Gerson recoveries, from conditions including melanoma, breast cancer, prostate cancer, bladder cancer, basal cell carcinoma and one young lady who recovered from severe epilepsy as the result of a nine month stint on the Gerson therapy.

From my own recovery experience, and close-up observations of a number of others who were on the therapy, I would offer a few suggestions for making life on the Gerson program go as smoothly as possible.

First, a suggestion about basic approach: If you are going to do it at all, completely give yourself to this very do-able metabolic cancer program. So many of us are tempted to hedge our bets, especially in the early stages when we are not feeling so great— you know, thoughts like: should I really be doing Gerson? How about Manner or Livingston or macrobiotics, instead? Maybe I should have done that chemo I was scheduled for after all, etc., etc. It was very helpful for me to come to a decision to be a 100% Gerson person, to pick one therapy and stick with it all the way.

Suggestion number two: no dietary exceptions. I did the whole diet, all day, every day, 365 days a year. No off-the-diet treats, ever — not on your birthday, Thanksgiving, Christmas, St. Swithins Day, or any other day you can think of for a "justified slip." When I got set in my mind in that stance, it made things nice and clear, and it had one interesting unanticipated side effect. On the big annual feast days, when the rest of the family was napping or tottering around sluggishly after the traditional turkey-stuffing-pie bash, I was the jolliest, most comfortable member of the clan.

Third suggestion: Homeopathic medicine works wonderfully well as an adjunct to the Gerson therapy. It does not interfere at all with the effectiveness of the program and is capable of providing major symptomatic relief and support. These remedies are now available in many health food stores. One excellent supplier is Biological Homeopathic Industries (BHI) in Albuquerque, NM.

Fourth suggestion: Regular chiropractic adjustments helped greatly to relieve physical tensions and tightness that accompanied body detoxification as the Gerson therapy did its healing work. It is important to find the right kind of chiropractor, one who is experienced, not too rough, and if possible one who is able to do cranial adjustments as well as working on the spine and neck.

Fifth suggestion: I made it a rule to avoid all unnecessary arguments, debates, and hassles, including minimizing my time in the company of people who lacked faith in the workability of the Gerson therapy, or in my chances of "making it." I was fortunate to be surrounded by family members and close friends who believed strongly in both the program and my outlook for success on it.

And last but not least: the Twelve Steps of Alcoholics Anonymous are not just for drunks. With their nonsectarian approach and their emphasis on "letting go and letting God," "one day at a time," and "easy does it," they are a great guide to serenity for anyone. They were my rule of life for the months I was on the therapy, and, as such, an absolute Godsend and life saver. It has been my observation that any recovering cancer patient's chances of sticking the course on the therapy go up about 100% when these principles, or their equivalent, are incorporated as part of the total recovery program.

PAULA PETERSON
COLON CANCER

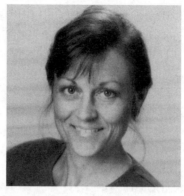

Greetings! Happiness and good health is our natural state — I am convinced of this. Doctors claimed that I would end up in a wheel chair for the rest of my life — that's how sick and weak I was as a child and young adult. There wasn't much hope for me, and I struggled for years with serious illness (including cancer), severe emotional depression, debilitating allergies and a collection of maladies that often accompany a suppressed immune system.

Not only do I consider my healing a miracle, I also consider my experience a life-saving blessing that I can pass onto others. Over 13 years ago, I was inspired to help others learn to increase their level of happiness, increase energy, feel better and heal themselves of serious illness just like I did. For many years, I offered a course in person, for groups in various public locations and in private homes. I offer information on-line at www.paulapeterson.com. My story is below and I think you may be surprised.

MY STORY:

Born with a life-threatening case of bronchial asthma and seriously debilitating allergies, I also struggled with severe emotional depression, a severely weakened immune system, a speech impediment, partial hearing loss in one ear, blurred vision, chronic fatigue, hypoglycemia and borderline diabetes, intestinal/colon cancer, PMS, weak knees and stiff, achy joints. I was allergic to many things: most foods, any animal with fur, hair or feathers, grass, pollen, fragrance, house dust, sensitivity to temperature fluctuations, etc. Eating only one peanut or a few soybeans would bring near death and a trip to the emergency hospital. It was a rare day when I was not sneezing, coughing and wheezing. I never knew a well day in my childhood and young adult years. Illness and depression was a way of life for me — I knew nothing else.

My immune system was so weak that I caught frequent colds and flu, several times a year. I was not able to be like other kids growing up. There was a lot of restriction and limits. The other kids in school never wanted me to be on their team during games since I was the *sickly kid*. The doctors claimed that I was in such a weakened condition that I would end up in a wheel chair for the rest of my life. I was so timid and ashamed of my disabilities that I could never look anyone in the eye.

I was on medication for years (which caused some long-term damage). Allergy desensitizing shots were administered every two days from childhood and throughout my young adult years. I could go nowhere without my breathalyzer. An asthma attack was always painful, frightening, exhausting and deeply discouraging. I never knew when an attack would occur. I was taken to emergency many times because I could not breathe, or I was in a near-death state of anaphylactic shock.

Needless to say, there were emotional instabilities and severe depression. This condition worsened as I entered puberty and young adulthood. Bouts with PMS each month laid me up in bed. Life was extremely difficult, but I managed to get married and hold down a full time job, even though both was always a struggle. I was exhausted most of the time, both physically and emotionally. My vision grew worse and I had to wear glasses or contact lenses at all times during waking hours. I began to have frequent toothaches. Needless to say, my marriage didn't last long.

Serious injuries from a motorcycle accident, and later a skiing accident, caused my knees to weaken: they often buckled without warning and were often stiff and achy. I also began to loose my hearing in one ear. Yes, I was a real mess! Luckily, I was cute and fortunate to be a straight-A student and later in my adult years, to go on to achieve a genius rating on the "Hardest IQ Test in the World" (not the highest genius rating but a genius rating, nevertheless!) — at least I had those attributes going for me.

My other attributes were determination, tenacity (stubbornness), an unquenchable thirst for knowledge and a strong faith in God. If I did not have those qualities to drive me, I would not be here today to tell my story — I would have long ago succumbed to my misery and illnesses and died an early death.

Thankfully, I not only recovered from ALL of the above ailments, I now enjoy a state of health, energy, happiness, enthusiasm for life and personal fulfillment that I never thought would ever be possible for me. If you were to compare the *old* me with the *new* me of today, you would hardly recognize that I am the same person. My mother tells me all too often how incredibly different and younger I look and behave. She is completely baffled.

REJUVENATION:

I no longer have asthma — not one trace of it. All of my allergies have disappeared (except for reactions to peanuts and soybeans). I happily enjoy all animal contact now. I sail through the *pollen season* with glee and no symptoms whatsoever. My immune system is now so strong that I rarely get colds and I never get the flu any more. Cancer tumors were eliminated through natural means. I can hike strenuous mountain trails with no breathing difficulties, no pain, no knee troubles and I no longer have stiff, achy joints. PMS completely disappeared. I threw away my glasses and contact lenses. Threw away all my medications, too.

My hearing returned to normal. Even though the speech impediment pops up only occasionally now, I went on to become a public speaker and presenter for many years and continue to do so.

My energy levels increased as my blood-sugar levels balanced out. My teeth are in great shape, never get yellow, never get plaque and there are no more toothaches (haven't been to a dentist in years). I have overcome and bypassed most of the so called *hereditary* diseases of my family (the type of disease and age that the disease usually occurs). All the female relatives in my family have had hysterectomies and other reproductive problems — not me! Surgeries for pancreas, stomach, colon, and gall bladder malfunctions, all of which are common in my family history, have not been an issue with me. And, since 1987, no more depression and no more emotional instabilities.

Is it any wonder that I emphasize living a life of gratitude and optimism?! My enthusiasm for life has grown and personal happiness has increased remarkably. I am so very grateful for all the experiences that led me to discover the healing methods, remedies and practices that pulled me through.

Because of the miracles in healing that occurred in my own life, it has become one of my most important missions: to share with others what I have learned and to be a source of encouragement, education and support for any level of improved health, well-being and attitude that folks desire to achieve for themselves.

The most effective part of my healing was determination, perseverance and faith in a Higher Power (God). This gave me the courage to leave behind unhealthy habits, such as in eating unhealthy foods and hanging out with unhealthy people.

First, I left unhealthy atmospheres behind, such as my family and friends who were frequently critical, unsupportive, close-minded, controlling and abusive. I began to *collect* healthier, more supportive friends.

I then began to change my diet, refining it again and again over the years. I stopped all medications and stopped going to the doctor who never supported me in choosing alternative measures, herbs, healthy food and alternative lifestyles as a method of healing.

I learned all I could, and still do, about healthy eating and healthy lifestyle. I cleansed my body and detoxified. Still do this periodically.

My faith in God kept me going no matter what. Faith in God has grown and deepened over the years and has proven to me over and over again that faith in and love of God gives me strength to accomplish all of the above.

IRENE STANANOUGHT
MALIGNANT MELANOMA

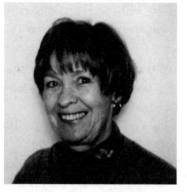

In March of 1996, I noticed my eyes became very yellow. A brown spot showed up on the inside of my left knee, followed by a black mole.

I visited my family doctor twice. He said the mole did not look serious. Four months later, I went for a general check up. My doctor looked at the mole and sent me to a specialist (Dr. J. Robert Madronich). On Nov. 18th, the mole was removed, biopsied, and diagnosed as modular malignant melanoma, Clarke's Level III. A second operation took place on Nov. 28th, 1996, a deep excision, and the report stated that "all malignancy was removed."

I was shocked when the mole was announced cancerous. I had never heard of melanoma before. I have always been health conscious and there is no family history of cancer in our family.

On a follow-up visit, the specialist informed me that I should come back every three months for a check-up and once per year for a chest x-ray. I asked, "Why do I have to come back every three months if you removed all the cancer, and why do I require a chest x-ray every year?" He said, "To see if the cancer had spread to the lymph nodes and the lungs." I asked, "How do I stop the cancer from spreading?"

He stated, "It's up to your immune system." I asked, "How do I improve my immune system?" He just looked at me and did not answer. That is when I decided to take my life into my own hands.

A few months prior to this I met a retired dentist who told me her story of a brain tumor 10 years earlier that was cured through diet and coffee enemas. She was an angel sent from heaven to save my life. I went to visit her and she told me about the Gerson Therapy and loaned me the book, *A Cancer Therapy*, by Dr. Max Gerson. She had also attended a couple of Charlotte's seminars.

I started reading Dr. Gerson's book at the same time I was feeling very tired and could not get rid of a flu and cold for about six weeks. After Christmas, I informed my family I was going to Mexico for the Gerson program. They were very sceptical and also did not realize the seriousness of the cancer.

I started on the 13 organic juices per day along with and the all organic diet and coffee enemas. Most of the flare ups (detoxification) happened during the first 18 months. The first year was the worst as my body detoxified. I had constant burning in various parts of my head. In July, 1997, I felt a tearing on the right lung and a year later a severe burning the same area. I think I may have passed a small tumor. It was ten months before my food started to digest. I remember the sweet odors after each coffee enema (DDT). Christmas, the following year I was really sick, almost passing out, I could hardly walk. The coffee enema on Christmas Eve finally released the chemicals from my liver, and after that night I stated to feel great. It is amazing the various areas of the body that required detoxification and healing.

When I was a child, we had a summer home where a neighbor sprayed the DDT twice a summer to control the bugs. My liver must have been overloaded with chemicals from DDT and the many other chemicals contained in food, etc. Also the many sun tanning days not realizing the dangers.

After the first year, I started to feel my body slowly growing stronger and healthier and my energy increased tremendously. My immune system has strengthened and I am not troubled by viruses. If I do get one, it is minor and gone quickly. When I first started the Gerson program, two years seemed forever. Now 5 1/2 years later, I feel better than I have for 20 years. I see Dr. Max Gerson becoming more recognized in many of the articles I read today.

I believe the most effective part of my healing was detoxifying, rebuilding the immune system, and staying with one method of healing. During the two years on the Gerson program I kept a journal and worked on releasing the many layers of past emotional trauma. I meditated every day, read every book on health and healing the body, and did yoga exercise, as well as walking. My family was supportive and lived with the two years of intense therapy. I could not have done this program if it wasn't for the support of my family.

I now see an excellent homeopathic doctor and continue eating only organic mostly vegetarian diet. I also try lead a less stressful, more simple lifestyle.

In June 2001, I revisited Doctor Melendez in Mexico for a 10 day detoxification and check up. All of the tumor markers came out below the normal range. This visit showed me that the body is capable of healing itself given the proper foods and detoxification and change of lifestyle. I recommend the Gerson Therapy to anyone.

AL SCHAEFER
COLON CANCER

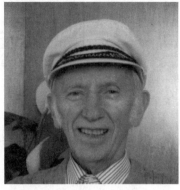

After testing positive on two pregnancy tests, I was convinced I was in a state of degeneration characteristic of cancer. Convinced, because previous information led me to believe that when a man (or a woman who is not pregnant) tests positive on a pregnancy tests, there are microbes within his system that are generating the hormone Chorionic Gonadotrophin. This hCG is the hormone of pregnancy. It was discovered by numerous researchers to be present in people with cancer. Dr. Virginia Livingston proved that a microbe present in a person with cancer produces this CG hormone. So, either I was pregnant or I was degenerated enough to be harboring the microbe, and maybe, a tumor somewhere in my body. You be the judge.

It was during the time my wife was suffering from the treatment for her breast cancer that we started looking for alternatives to the conventional methods. After her death, I continued searching for the explanation for why she got cancer and why the doctors did nothing but mutilate her body without slowing or stopping the progress of the cancer. I felt betrayed by medicine of the USA. Many sources tried to explain carcinogenesis, but only one resonated with my reasoning; the one Dr. Virginia Livingston gave.

This understanding of the microbial basis of cancer clearly defined the enemy as being a microbe whose excretion warded off the immune system by faking it out. The same hormone keeps the embryo from being attack by the immune system. Not only did Dr. Virginia provide a means to detect a cancerous degeneration early, but she provided a nutritional program to recover. All this meant no mutilation to me, and the ultimate alternative to the mutilation of conventional methods.

The refrain "If only I had known before" accompanied the sobs of regret, for my wife's tortuous life and death resulting from cancer and the conventional doctor's treatment, and for the betrayal by my idol in the form of doctors of medicine. After the sobbing, anger welled up, expressing itself in my imagination of how to get even. Indeed, it was a refrain, after each new finding.

If only we had known before, we would have abandoned the conventional, palliative methods, and used a nutritional program for her recovery. I believe Dorothy, my wife of 22 years, would be alive today if the 2 surgeries, 33 radiations and 7 chemos hadn't killed her. Her last words to me were, "They don't know what they are doing." During this horrible betrayal she prayed that, "A cure be found so others do not have to suffer like I am." The refrain, and this prayer, keep ruminating in my mind, "If only I had known before."

At the beginning of our search we found Laetrile IV injections did relieve her pain, but didn't slow the descent. A more inclusive program was required which we didn't know, learning later there is no magic bullet. The Laetrile program with pancreatic enzymes and stomach enzymes, along with massive doses of emulsified Vitamin A, plus vegetarian diet are called for early after diagnosis. Too late for Laetrile to ward off her death 16 months after diagnosis.

Once my emotions settled, I made her prayer my goal. It has motivated me since then, hoping to help others search for the way to stay healthy, instead of regretting "If only I had known before." This goal consumes me. My grief, anger and this goal melded into the activities of the local chapter of the Cancer Victors and Friends, of which I was elected their president. Through the attendees, I could empathize with their grieving, channel my anger, believing that the people who chose alternatives were taking business from the oncologist, and fulfill her prayer by informing others of my new-found options. This search for information was a magnet. The studies led me to scheduling speakers for the chapter's monthly meetings. The more I learned the more I searched, and the more time I spent, even at the expense of my sleep, to uncover what I did not know before. I kept this pace for 2 1/2 years after her death. I found the cure for cancer in the literature, and many did not suffer like she did, because they followed the authors for recovery, and avoided radiation and chemo. Her prayer was being answered, while its pursuit depleted my energies to the braking point.

Now, the crossroads. I learned how to cure cancer. I learned how to get cancer. The latter wasn't in the literature. The unrelenting search of the literature into the wee hours, the scheduling of monthly speakers and monthly board meetings along with the grief and anger taught me the components required to get cancer. My energy got up and went. I was tired in the afternoon and started drinking coffee. The color of my skin became colorless, like this paper. Now, I had to change directions.

The avid search of the literature and the speakers told about non-invasive tests for this condition of degeneration associated with cancer, and cancer cure. Sure? The scientist in me said, "Now it is time to test the hypothesis. If this unconventional, far-out stuff proves out, I can testify (like I am doing now). If it's fake, my death will also be testimony (not quite so loud)." I put the burden on God. "If I give my body Your nutrients, the things that will not harm it, as I believe You intended, then I believe You will bless this venture." The flip side of this is that I had already vowed, publicly, that, "If I ever get cancer I will not take the conventional route. I would rather die." This declaration followed on the heels of my Dorothy's horrible experience, in the heat of the battle, so to speak. But, 2 1/2 years after her death the decision was coldly scientific, relying on the integrity of the researchers. I shout that declaration even more loudly, now, as I look back. So, let's see if these non-invasive tests are any good?

This scientist started testing the hypothesis. Over Christmas holiday, 1977, I flew to the Freeport, Bahamas, to have Lawrence Burton's test with his cancer marker. He told me, "You have an old tumor that is breaking up." I wanted his test, but not his program. I had long ago decided that I would use the Max Gerson program to get well. It was more in keeping with "Do No Harm." Back home I sent a urine specimen to Dr. Navarro in the Philippines, to test for that hormone of pregnancy (CG). His letter asked, "Where is your old tumor." I needed a little more confirmation. I convinced my Osteopathic doctor to write a prescription for a CG test. "What, do you think you're pregnant, Al?" BioScience Lab's (Van Nuys, CA) test showed positive, indicating three possibilities of cancer or pregnancy. Wow! Here this lab confirmed that the CG indicated cancer in three cases. They didn't know about Dr. Virginia's finding. These three tests, and my gut feeling, convinced me. Get more serious, Al. At the end of May, 1978, I went to the Livingston Clinic, in San Diego. There, 3 more tests substantiated that the CG and Burton's test were good. The darkfield exam of my blood showed a multitude of strange microbes, just like Dr. Virginia had said. I saw them with my own eyes. My liver function tests were askew. The CEA (Carcino Embryonic Antigen), a standard, conventional test for colon cancer, read 74. (Greater than 5 signals danger, more than 10 warns of metastasis, per Merck Manual.) Dr. Virginia wanted to do an exploratory to confirm with a biopsy. I stuck by my vow. Besides I learned that biopsy is unreliable at least 25% of the time. Six tests confirmed the hypothesis that there are non-invasive tests for degeneration, without biopsy.

When I told Dr. Virginia I was going to the Gerson clinic for the nutritional program, she put her arm around my shoulder and said, "You are making a wise choice Mr. Schaefer. Bless you." After leaving the Gerson clinic, I returned to the Livingston Clinic. Virginia was excited about the vigor of my red blood cells, without those pesky, superfluous microbes. Both of us were happy.

Now to test the *Cure* hypothesis.

The program I followed is clearly spelled out on page 236 of the Max Gerson book, *A Cancer Therapy*. By the time my 20-day stay was over was I realized I had reversed the decline, cleaned out the detrimental microbes and was on the road to recovery. The rest would be the tough part — to rebuild a degenerate body. The hCG went to zero, then bounced to high normal. Liver function tests bounced around until 2 years later, when they normalized. When I entered I weighed 125 lbs. Went to 115. Before I left I started gaining weight. After a couple months at home, I weighed in at a husky 147 lbs. I could not hold to the strict program once at home as I worked full time, but the program was working. Cure hypothesis confirmed!

The Livingston Clinic makes a vaccine to stir the immune system against the detrimental microbes. When I first checked in I donated some urine. While I was at Gerson, the lab made a vaccine from my hCG-generating microbes. Upon my return I picked up the vaccine and headed home.

Experiments complete.

Time for evaluation: The best, readily available blood test for hCG is a Radio-immuno Assay for hCG beta subunit, quantitative. Standard labs can do this test. Darkfield test is done in a doctors office provided he has a darkfield condenser for his microscope and knows how to read what he sees.

From what I learned: There is no one component in the Gerson program that is more important than the other. Since then, I have learned that other researchers have verified the importance of each of these components. Other nutrition programs use the Gerson program as a starter, modifying it to accommodate meek patients and the clinic's resources.

In the past 20 years, I have conversed with many cancer patients and facilitated support groups, still in pursuit of Dorothy's prayer. Observation and conclusions came naturally. Early detection is paramount, especially if determined by non-invasive tests like the hCG. Success with the nutritional programs depends on the state of depletion of the patient. The more depleted the person's body, the steeper the climb, and longer the journey to recovery. All conventional treatments increase the depletion. If the person is young, under 40 to 45, chances improve. Each individual is not a statistic. Sheer determination, asking for God's help, plays a major role in recovery in spite of the previous degeneration. For me, it's been a great scientific experiment! A great adventure! Other survivors have concurred.

In quiet sadness, I regret not having known all this before. My Dorothy's sacrifice has saved the lives of many cancer patients. May this testimony suffice for you.

Patty Saccoman
Breast Cancer

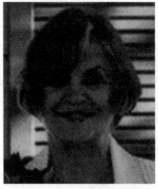

At age 64, I was surprised when I noticed a lump in my right breast. A mother of six, grandmother of twelve, and great-grandmother of three, I led an active life. An ultrasound in August 1997 revealed a suspicious mass. When imaged with mammography in October 1997, it was 15x15x20-mm and was a suspected cancer growth. I was diagnosed with ductile carcinoma that month. My doctor hypothesized that the cancer had begun growing about 8 years prior to its appearance. That had be a time of stress for me, and I believe stress was the prime factor in the cancer's development.

My doctor was very concerned that the cancer had metastasized, and he recommended a comprehensive exam including a biopsy. The cancer had not spread at this point, but the biopsy revealed a malignant tumor. My doctor proposed two courses of action, either a total mastectomy or a lumpectomy with removal of the lymph nodes under my arm followed by aggressive radiation. He gave me a death sentence. It has now been six years since then and I am still cancer free. I wanted to keep my lymph nodes and wanted to start with the least invasive treatment options first. I chose a lumpectomy. The doctor was shocked that I didn't want my lymph nodes removed. When I arrived for the surgery, he refused to do the lumpectomy, because I would not authorize removal of the lymph nodes.

The surgeon referred me to oncologist who tried to scare me into doing not only the lumpectomy, but also total removal of the lymph nodes under my arm. I was anxious after my visit because my doctor was so aggressive. He told me that if he were my husband, he would duct tape my mouth shut and force me to have the radical surgery. That was the last time I went to that doctor! After that, I decided to forego the lumpectomy altogether and continue to look for alternative therapies.

My husband and I went to a medical symposium where I met an old friend who recommended supplementing with Haelan, a fermented soy beverage. I also met Joe Todesco, whose company manufactures and imports Haelan. After several hours, I agreed that Haelan was worth a try.

I started drinking a bottle per day of Haelan on November 4, 1997. I had a follow-up mammogram six weeks later that revealed a significant decrease in tumor size. My doctor was amazed. A third mammogram revealed a 50% reduction in the vessel supplying nutrients to the tumor. I had four mammograms and each time the tumor was measured, it had decreased in size.

I believe the most effective part of my healing was drinking Haelan and my strong faith in God. I believe my cancer was a call, an opportunity to be thankful for every second of my life!

I will celebrate my 70th birthday in March of 2003. I praise God from whom all blessings flow, and thank my loving husband and family for their support.

BOB BELL

SQUAMOUS CELL CARCINOMA

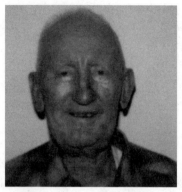

It all started June 1996, when a type of cancer called squamous cell carcinoma, like skin cancer, was discovered at the base of my tongue on the left side. This is very common in people who smoke or chew tobacco. But I have never done either of these, and it was a surprise to the medical establishment.

It was decided that surgery was the best procedure. An operation was performed at UCSF. The doctor cut the skin from my lip, down under my jaw and back up to the ear. Then the skin was lifted up and the jaw removed so he could get to the tongue. The doctor then removed one-third of my tongue along with the cancer tumor and confirmed that he got all of the cancer. Then he took a muscle out of my chest to put into my cheek to keep the cheek from sinking in.

After 2 weeks stay in the hospital, I continued check-ups with the doctor at UCSF every three months to make sure the cancer was not returning.

In January 2000, on one of my check ups, it was discovered that the tumor had come back and the doctor suggested another radical operation would be the only way to remove it. I refused to do another operation. I also refused to do any radiation or chemotherapy and opted to find an alternative procedure somewhere. Lucky for me — I found Dr. Phillip Minton in Reno, Nevada who does alternative treatments with infusing, natural products.

I started alternative care which included homeopathic, immune and detoxifying by infusion, for an initial three week period. This was followed by injections near the tumor three times a week for a couple of months. I would have been very happy just to keep the tumor from growing any larger, but the doctor and I were pleasantly surprised to find out the tumor was shrinking and eventually disappeared completely. Upon taking PET scans and MRI's, all signs showed that the tumor was gone and any other cancer in the neck area was non-existent.

Naturally, there is no guarantee that the cancer will not come back, but so far I am cancer free. I do know if the cancer does come back, I will only follow the alternative treatments that proved so well in eradicating the cancer tumor that I had.

My only regret is that I did not know or explore the type of alternative treatment prior to the radical surgery, as that surgery did leave my face, tongue and jaw disfigured.

If you need any more information, or want me to amplify any of these statements, please contact me, and I will gladly give you more detail.

Thank you for letting my story out as it may help someone else.

OLIVIA DE HAULLEVILLE
BREAST CANCER

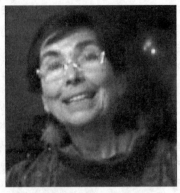

My Stage 2 breast cancer was discovered in the Spring of 1999, after a biopsy revealed two estrogen-receptive DCIS growths in my left breast, one the size of a pea. Radical mastectomy was immediately recommended. Several *second opinions* also recommended that I should have the 'offending breast' totally removed, including the lymph node which would determine whether chemotherapy and/or radiation would be needed. I was also prescribed Tamoxifen.

However, I refused all of these options. I immediately changed my diet to eliminate all estrogen foods, i.e. milk and meat products, which have received hormone additives. I stayed clear of the microwaves, increased my already mostly Asian diet of seaweed, mushrooms and tofu, and took larger doses of vitamins and supplements.

Being a Holistic Practitioner (Clinical Hypnotherapist), I realized the importance of an integrative approach. My original doctor, Yeshi Dhonden (previous doctor to H.H. The Dalai Lama) supplied me with Tibetan herbal pills, but since I failed to establish a good connection between Tibetan and Western medicine, I decided to forego this initial treatment after my supply was exhausted.

Shortly after, I was lucky enough to be present at a lecture by Albert Sanchez on Poly-MVA. I was so impressed by this man that I failed to take notice of the extensive testimonials he offered on this product. I decided instead to purchase Dr. M. Garnett's personal journal: *First Pulse.* I read this book with fascination! Being dedicated to a natural way of life, I was able to discern the power in this substance immediately and immediately had it checked out by my Tibetan doctor who gave me the go ahead.

In July 1999, in order to convince me of the urgency of a mastectomy, my oncologist requested another mammogram. In fact, the mammogram was done twice… but still could show no suspicious results! My oncologist seemed non-plussed. He asked me what I proposed to do next; without hesitation I answered: "Continue the Poly-MVA."

Index
by Leonard S. Rosenbaum